U0339564

生育力保护

——宫内疾病诊治流程 及手术操作规范

主 审 冯力民 薛 敏

主 编 李雪英

本书由湖南省卫健委
技术创新项目经费资助出版

CTS K 湖南科学技术出版社 · 长沙

编委会

序

  现代化的中国医疗最大的问题就是非同质化，其原因是我们地域辽阔，人口众多，而医生的需求量非常大，不同层次的医生有着不同的医学背景、不同的专科背景、不同的培训背景，所以才造成我们医疗质量的非同质化。在全世界信息化的进程中，患者会掌握更多的医学信息，并对自己的病情有更多、更深刻地了解。在这种情况下，更要求我们的医生对疾病能做出正确判断，选择最恰当的治疗方法，和对疾病未来的走向有很好的预测，这样才能真正提高我们的医疗质量。患者仅知道疾病的"今天"，而我们会评判各种治疗的利弊，预见疾病的走向。

  对于宫内疾病的诊断和治疗，全世界都处于一种不断高度重视的状态，其原因何在呢？2019 年的欧洲妇科内镜学会（ESGE）会上，美国一位著名的生殖医生在大会演讲时谈到，去生殖中心寻求辅助生育帮助的 40 岁以上的女性已经超过了 25%。由此可见，宫内疾病的诊断和治疗对于子宫来说，保留其生育的能力越来越被需要和重视。

  李雪英主任领衔全国的专家共同书写了这本《生育力保护——宫内疾病诊治流程及手术操作规范》，涵盖九大类疾病的治疗规范和护理规范，包括了致死并发症的讲解和宫内疾病的病理学理论，最重要的还有近年全球七大宫内疾病指南的解读。这本规范把宫内疾病诊治同质化跃然纸上，一本小小的口袋书能让我们按照疾病指南和专家共识，做出最正确的诊疗。这是为宫内疾病诊治同质化的进程做出有益的贡献，开卷有益，让大家在宫内疾病的诊疗路上安全前行！

2023 年 8 月 6 日

前　言

　　宫腔镜技术是近30年高速发展的微创技术，宫腔镜之母夏恩兰教授把宫腔镜技术在我国近30年的发展分为三个阶段：第一个阶段（1990—2000年）惊艳全国，第二阶段（2000—2010年）星火燎燃，第三阶段（2010年至今）遍地开花。

　　湖南省妇幼保健院（以下简称我院）2000年在星火燎燃阶段开始开展宫腔镜技术，从最简单的宫腔镜检查开始，这20多年在全体从事宫腔镜研究医师的共同努力下，我院宫腔镜技术得到飞速发展。近10年来，每年宫腔镜检查及手术近万例；2014年湖南省妇幼保健与优生优育协会宫内疾病防治专业委员会成立并挂靠我院；2015年我院成立了湖南省首个宫内疾病示范病房；2017年成为湖南省首个宫内疾病防治建设项目示范医院和培训中心。

　　我有幸从2013年宫腔镜技术遍地开花的阶段开始学习宫腔镜技术，在学习的过程中得益于崔超美主任的指导和冯力民教授无私教诲，以及前辈们学术的交流与分享，我开始深深地热爱宫腔镜技术，并得到不断成长。近10年湖南省宫腔镜技术也和全国各地一样蓬勃发展，大部分县级医院都逐步开展了宫腔镜技术。夏恩兰老师说"小宫腔，大世界"，宫腔是女性生命的摇篮。随着生育政策放开，保护宫腔，保护育龄女性的生育功能成了我们妇产科医师义不容辞的责任，因此宫内疾病诊治从初学者开始就需要规范化，制订一套临床实用的宫内疾病诊治流程和手术操作规范，给初学者或者基层医师参考，在临床实践中按照规范实施，对保护患者的宫腔和子宫内膜是非常必要的。2018年，我科申请了湖南省创新项目《利用微无创技术保护育龄女性的生育功能》；2019年，我院制定了《生育力保护——宫内疾病诊治流程和手术操作规范》，邀请冯力民教授及湖南省相关专家进行讨论并修改形成初稿编辑成册，在湖南省宫内疾病诊治培训班作为培训资料。此后有不少初学者希望得到这本培训资料，于是萌生了出版的想法并得到了冯力民教授的鼓励。在冯力民教授精心指导下，我们用半年时间进行反复地修改和完善，并配上了一些手术视频课程供初学者参考。不足之处欢迎大家不吝赐教，可发送邮件至1620712527@qq.com，对我们的工作予以批评指正，以期再次修订进一步完善。

在本书出版之际，我代表编写团队感谢冯力民教授和薛敏教授的大力支持、鼓励与肯定！感谢中南大学湘雅医院张怡教授、刘惠宁教授，中南大学湘雅二医院张洪文教授、湖南省妇幼保健院方超英教授在初稿形成中提出宝贵意见及建议，感谢全体编委的辛苦付出！感谢湖南省妇幼保健与优生优育协会的大力支持！本书出版经费由湖南省创新项目资助。

李雪英

2023 年 8 月 12 日

|目 录|

第一章　子宫内膜息肉的诊治流程及技术规范

　　子宫内膜息肉（endometrial polyp，EP）是在子宫内膜表面突出的良性结节，是由子宫内膜腺体及含厚壁血管的纤维化子宫内膜间质构成的突出于子宫内膜表面的良性结节，是常见的子宫内膜病变之一，可引起异常子宫出血与不孕，可恶变。35 岁以下的女性子宫内膜息肉的发病率约为 3％，35 岁以上的女性约为 23％，绝经后妇女的发病率最高，约为 31％，高峰年龄为 50 岁，70 岁以后很少发生。而在不孕患者中，子宫内膜息肉的患病率增加明显，其确切发生率难以确定，与所用检查手段有关，据报道为 2.8％～34.9％。目前中国妇女子宫内膜息肉发病率不断提高，为 24％～25％。若息肉体积较为细小，患者在临床发病时并不会出现明显症状，但在其不断地增长后，则会导致患者发生子宫异常出血或是出现血性阴道分泌物等情况，对患者的身体健康造成较大影响。尤其是子宫内膜息肉可能会导致不孕，对患者的身心健康有较大影响。

一、诊断

　　1. 临床表现：有月经量增多、经间期出血、经期延长、不规则子宫出血或不孕等病症。

　　2. 体格检查：妇科检查可无异常，或宫颈外口处看到或触及息肉。

　　3. 影像学检查：超声提示宫内稍高回声团块，或内膜回声不均匀，局部回声增强。

　　4. 宫腔镜检查：可见子宫内膜表面突出的良性结节，表面光滑，常有血管，可单发或多发，大小不一，形态多样。

5. 病理检查：将取出的组织或切除的息肉送病检以明确诊断，并鉴别子宫黏膜下肌瘤、功能失调性子宫出血及子宫内膜癌等病变。

二、鉴别诊断

1. 子宫黏膜下肌瘤：多有阴道分泌物多、经量多、经期长、不规则子宫出血或不孕症状。妇科检查子宫大小可正常，黏膜下肌瘤脱出于宫颈口可见质地中等赘生物，超声提示宫腔内低回声肿块，边界清，有包膜。

2. 子宫内膜癌：主要表现为阴道流血或阴道排液，病灶累及宫颈可出现宫腔积脓、下腹疼痛等。早期妇科检查无异常，晚期可有子宫增大，合并宫腔积脓时可有明显压痛。超声提示宫腔内不均质区，或宫腔线消失，肌层内不均匀回声区。

三、治疗

（一）观察（期待治疗）

6.3%～27%绝经前无症状子宫内膜息肉（直径＜1 cm）可于1年内自然消退。因此，对于无症状、无恶变高危因素、息肉直径＜1 cm 的绝经前子宫内膜息肉患者，可观察随访。期待治疗推荐3～6个月超声复检1次，若病情稳定，则可每年随诊1次，若息肉增大或出现症状则需要进一步治疗。

（二）药物治疗

药物治疗很少单独用于治疗子宫内膜息肉，一般用于异常子宫出血患者宫腔镜检查术前，鉴别真性息肉与假性息肉，或术后预防子宫内膜息肉复发及恶变，对于存在恶变高危因素的患者，需排除息肉恶变后再行药物治疗。常用药物包括孕激素类药物、复方口服避孕药（combined oral contraceptive，COC）等。合并慢性子宫内膜炎患者，可给予抗生素治疗。

（三）手术治疗

1. 适应证：①有症状的息肉，表现为经量增多、经期延长、经间期出血、同房出血、不孕症、绝经后出血等；②直径＞10 mm 的息肉；③怀疑恶变，或存在恶变高危因素，如年龄＞60 岁，绝经状态，肥胖，糖尿病，高血压，使用他莫昔芬；④绝经后无症状息肉。

2. 麻醉方式：①静脉全麻；②硬膜外或区域阻滞麻醉；③全身麻醉。

3. 手术时机：①月经后 2～7 天内视野最清晰，尽量避开月经前期；②本次月经周期无性生活；③如因经期延长就诊可选月经第 7 天后，如无规律月经，血净后可考虑手术；④有不可控出血时可急诊手术。

4. 术前准备：①病情告知与知情同意。②宫颈准备：术前晚酌情放置宫颈扩张棒扩张宫颈或阴道上药［米索前列醇 0.4 mg 或卡孕栓 1 mg（排除米索前列醇禁忌证）］软化宫颈，手术开始前 10 分钟静脉给予间苯三酚软化宫颈的效果也较好。③绝经时间长、子宫及子宫颈萎缩严重患者的子宫颈预处理用雌激素，可增加萎缩阴道、子宫及子宫颈的结缔组织弹性，促进组织增生，有助于子宫颈软化松弛。④术前禁食 6 小时以上。

5. 手术操作规范：

（1）宫腔镜电切术：单极及双极电切技术均可安全有效地应用于子宫内膜息肉手术，部分研究显示，双极手术因使用等渗液体，灌流液过吸收发生率低，手术时间更短；而单极器械则更为普及，价格更低。

1）患者取膀胱截石位，静脉全身麻醉后，常规消毒铺巾。探查宫腔深度后，利用扩宫器扩张子宫颈至 7 号。

2）置入宫腔检查镜，全面探查宫颈及宫腔情况，明确息肉位置、大小及数量，宫角及双侧输卵管开口情况。

3）再次宫颈扩张器扩张宫颈至 10 号（根据具体电切器械决定），置入宫腔镜电切镜，在直视下以环状电极（切割功率为 280 W，电凝功率为 80 W）从息肉游离端向根蒂部连续切除，当息肉位置特殊时可使用特殊的电切环，如直角环切割可较精确地在视野范围内进行组织切除，防止切割过深，可有效处理蒂部位于子宫底或输卵管开口处的息肉。对于无蒂息肉，可以先不通电，当完全暴露出息肉底部时再激活电循环。这样可尽量减少对于子宫壁的任何热损伤及降低穿孔风险。基底部出血可用电凝止血，手术中注意勿伤及子宫肌层及息肉周边的子宫内膜，保护内膜基底层。

4）术后全面探查宫腔息肉切除是否干净，有无活动性出血，确定息肉彻底清除且无活动性出血后结束手术。

（2）冷刀系统：

1）宫腔镜刨削系统：目前国内常应用的宫腔镜电动刨削系统，包括一次性 MyoSure（美奥舒）和 IBS（Integrated Bigatti Shaver）系统，均为机械冷刀切割宫腔组织、粉碎和移除系统，其工作原理是通过刨削刀头在切割窗内高速旋转往复完成组织的机械切割，同时通过负压将切除的组织快速吸引排出宫腔，其优势在于显著减少了器械进出宫腔的次数，提高手术效率，缩短手术时间，且过程不产生热量，无热损伤风险。

①取膀胱截石位，静脉麻醉后，常规消毒铺巾，探查宫腔深度后，扩张宫颈至 7 号。

②置入宫腔镜行宫腔镜检查，再次确认宫腔形态、内膜情况，息肉的位置、大小和数量，宫角及双侧输卵管开口情况。

③宫腔组织机械性旋切装置的真空负压，根据膨宫液的进出平衡原则设定在 250～350 mmHg（33.3～46.7 kPa）之间，膨宫机压力需设定在 80～100 mmHg（10.7～13.3 kPa），流速调至 500 mL/min。如为一次性宫腔组织切除装置，可不需要扩张宫颈，如为 IBS 刨削系统，需要用扩宫器扩张宫颈至 10 号。

④经宫腔镜工作通道插入组织切除装置进行手术操作。将机械性宫腔组织旋切装置的切割窗直接紧贴息肉表面，在息肉表面来回"扫"，当接近息肉根部时，切除装置的切割窗最好距离根部 3～5 mm，或者将切割窗稍偏向一侧，利用该器械的负压吸引作用，吸引息肉基底部的组织进入切割窗进行切割，避免切割窗正面紧贴息肉基底部旋转切割时损伤息肉根部下方的内膜及肌层。检查息肉完全切除干净遂停止手术。

2）宫腔镜微型器械切除术：指宫腔镜下应用显微剪刀或抓钳等微型器械切除息肉。

①取膀胱截石位，静脉麻醉后，常规消毒铺巾，探查宫腔深度后，扩张宫颈至 7 号。

②缓慢置入宫腔镜，宫腔镜下仔细检查宫颈、宫腔，对息肉进行定位，确定息肉大小和数量数目，宫角及双侧输卵管开口情况。

③在目标息肉根蒂处打开抓钳，再轻轻合上抓钳，用钳夹夹住息肉后向患者头端推，判断根蒂径线后并向一个方向扭转，直至息肉与宫壁完全分离，然后将游离的息肉从宫腔取出。或者用微型剪刀从息肉蒂部剪断，完整地摘除息肉。

不同宫腔镜息肉去除技术的临床结果没有显著差异（C 级）。

6. 术中术后注意事项：

（1）严格按照手术操作规程要求，实施无菌操作，排空气体，动作轻柔，预防子宫穿孔及周围脏器损伤、出血、感染、气体栓塞等发生；术中一旦发现子宫穿孔，立即停止操作，并注射宫缩剂促进子宫收缩，避免组织嵌顿及脏器损伤。根据穿孔器械、是否有继发损伤做相应处理。

（2）术中注意子宫黏膜下肌瘤和息肉鉴别。主要的宫腔镜下鉴别特征是子宫内膜息肉：柔软可随着膨宫液体的流动而摆动，宫腔镜镜体头部轻轻进入息肉内，而黏膜下肌瘤质地硬，不随膨宫液体的流动而摆动，镜体不能插入黏膜下肌瘤内。

（3）宫腔镜术中操作尽量保护子宫内膜，电切术中注意识别内膜功能层及肌层。如为功能层，电切术中可见典型的散在白色点状腺体，子宫肌层则为致密的纵横交错的网状纤维结构，看不到点状腺体组织。术中切除息肉蒂部时注意不要伤及子宫内膜基底层和息肉周边的内膜组织，以免引起子宫内膜损伤导致宫腔粘连；对于有宫腔粘连风险的病人，建议术后利用宫腔内留置球囊和注射透明质酸钠凝胶的方法，以减少术后的宫腔粘连。

（四）术后长期管理

1. 青春期：缺乏相关的临床数据研究，关注子宫内膜息肉的高危因素并进行治疗，恢复正常月经周期，预防复发。

2. 育龄期：有生育要求者在子宫内膜息肉切除术后应尽快妊娠，近期无生育要求者以药物治疗预防息肉复发为主，包括孕激素、复方口服避孕药、左炔诺孕酮宫内缓释节育系统（levonorgestrel-releasing intrauterine system，LNG-IUS）；无生育要求者应综合治疗，包括药物治疗、定期随访、健康教育及药物不良作用的管理。

3. 围绝经期：初始治疗的彻底性，切割深度需达子宫内膜基底层，术后需要孕激素治疗调整月经周期，或者 LNG-IUS 放置至绝经。

4. 绝经后：健康宣教，定期随访。

（五）诊治流程（图1－1）

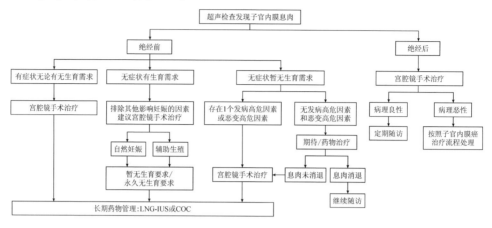

图1－1　子宫内膜息肉诊治流程

吴岭　李雪英

【参考文献】

［1］黄丽华，向梅. 子宫内膜息肉研究新进展［J］. 国际妇产科学杂志，2014，41（1）：43－46.

［2］林红娣，余幼芬，沈军英. 宫腔镜下刮宫术与电切术治疗子宫内膜息肉的疗效及对妊娠结局影响［J］. 中国妇幼保健，2018，33（4）：921－923.

［3］张旭垠，华克勤. 子宫内膜息肉治疗后预防复发策略［J］. 中国实用妇科与产科杂志，2016，32（11）：1079－1082.

［4］孙东岩，王燕，姚冬梅，等. 美奥舒组织切除系统治疗功能良性占位病变临床分析［J］. 现代妇产科进展，2017，26（6）：463－467.

［5］冯力民. 子宫内膜息肉的手术治疗［J］. 中国实用妇科与产科杂志，2022，38（3）：269－272.

［6］American Association of Gynecologic Laparoscopists. AAGL practice report：practice guidelines for the diagnosis and management of endometrial polyps［J］. J Minim Invasive Gynecol，2012，19（1）：3－10.

［7］PEREIRA N，PETRINI A C，LEKOVICH J P，et al. Surgical management of endometrial polyps in infertile women：a comprehensive review［J］. Surg Res Pract，2015，2015：914－390.

［8］American Association of Gynecologic Laparoscopists［J］. J Minim Invasive Gynecol. 2012 Jan—Feb；19（1）：3—10.

［9］VAN DONGEN H，EMANUEL M H，WOLTERBEEK R，et al. Hysteroscopic morcellator for removal of intrauterine polyps and myomas：a randomized controlled pilot study among residents in training［J］. J Minim Invasive Gynecol，2008，15（4）：466—471.

［10］陈澜，杨旖赛，何晓英，等. 子宫内膜息肉的长期管理［J］. 中国计划生育和妇产科，2021，13（7）：20—22.

［11］中国优生科学协会生殖道疾病诊治分会，中国医师协会微无创医学专业委员会妇科肿瘤学组. 子宫内膜息肉诊治中国专家共识（2022年版）［J］. 中国实用妇科与产科杂志，2022，38（8）：809—813.

［12］中华医学会妇产科学分会妇科内镜学组. 宫腔镜手术子宫颈预处理临床实践指南［J］. 中华妇产科杂志，2020，55（12）：813—817.

［13］全佳丽，冯力民，薛凤霞，等. 子宫内膜息肉临床诊疗路径［J］. 中华妇产科杂志，2022，57（7）：491—495.

第二章 子宫黏膜下肌瘤的 诊治流程及手术操作规范

子宫肌瘤是子宫平滑肌组织增生而形成的良性肿瘤，是女性最常见的良性肿瘤。子宫肌瘤的发病率难以准确统计，估计育龄期妇女的患病率可达 25%，根据尸体解剖统计的发病率可达 50% 以上。子宫肌瘤根据其与子宫肌壁的解剖学关系分为黏膜下肌瘤、肌壁间肌瘤和浆膜下肌瘤，与肌壁间和浆膜下肌瘤相比，黏膜下肌瘤的发病率仅占总体发病率的 5.5%~16.6%。但是，由于黏膜下肌瘤生长在子宫腔内或凸向子宫腔生长，则更容易引起异常子宫出血和（或）妊娠失败，即使是少数能够妊娠的患者，其流产、早产和孕产期病率亦会明显上升。

一、诊断

1. 临床表现：有经量增多、经期延长等异常子宫出血，白带增多，阴道排液，不孕等病症。

2. 体格检查：妇科检查可发现子宫稍增大或正常大小，个别肌瘤有蒂部脱入宫颈甚至阴道内。

3. 影像学检查：超声提示子宫低回声肿块，向宫腔突出，包膜完整，边界清楚，内膜线前移或后移。

4. 宫腔镜检查：可见子宫内有单个或多个肌性凸起结节，表面光滑，可有蒂部或仅向宫腔内突出。宫腔镜下黏膜下子宫肌瘤分类：0 型（有蒂黏膜下肌瘤，宫腔镜下见肌瘤有一个蒂与宫腔相连）；Ⅰ 型（无蒂黏膜下肌瘤，向肌层扩展≤50%，宫腔镜下见肌瘤与宫壁成一个<90°的夹角）；Ⅱ 型（无蒂黏膜下肌瘤，向肌层扩展>50%，宫腔镜下见肌瘤与宫壁成一个>90°的夹角）。

5. 病理检查：将取出的组织或切除的肌瘤送病检，提示平滑肌瘤。

二、鉴别诊断

1. 子宫内膜息肉：多表现为经量增多、经期延长或经间期出血，妇科检查子宫正常大小或有赘生物脱出于宫颈口，超声提示宫腔内稍高回声光团，回声不均匀，宫腔镜检和病检可明确诊断。

2. 子宫腺肌病：可有子宫增大、月经增多等。局限型子宫腺肌病类似子宫肌壁间肌瘤，质硬。但子宫腺肌病继发性痛经明显，子宫多呈均匀增大，超声检查及外周血 CA125 检测有助于诊断，但有时两者可以并存。

3. 子宫内膜癌：主要表现为阴道流血或阴道排液，病灶累及宫颈可出现宫腔积脓、下腹疼痛等。早期妇科检查无异常，晚期可有子宫增大，合并宫腔积脓时可有明显压痛。超声提示宫腔内不均质区，或宫腔线消失，肌层内不均质回声区，需病理检查确诊。

三、治疗

（一）手术指征

任何影响子宫腔或子宫颈管正常解剖学形态、伴发异常子宫出血、不孕等病症的子宫肌瘤均应考虑手术。

1. 0 型黏膜下肌瘤。

2. Ⅰ～Ⅱ型黏膜下肌瘤，肌瘤直径≤5.0 cm。

3. 肌壁间肌瘤向子宫腔生长，宫腔面肌瘤覆盖肌层组织≤0.5 cm，浆膜面肌层组织≥0.5 cm。

4. 各类脱入阴道的子宫或宫颈黏膜下肌瘤。

5. 子宫腔长度≤12 cm。

6. 子宫体积<8～10 周妊娠大小。

7. 排除肌瘤恶变。

8. Ⅲ型黏膜下肌瘤担心日后肌瘤太大无法行宫腔镜手术者，或者 IVF-ET（体外受精－胚胎移植）前准备担心妊娠后肌瘤长大压迫宫内膜者，可酌情考虑宫腔镜手术。但Ⅲ型黏膜下肌瘤是否行宫腔镜切除需结合肌瘤大小、位置及术者水平酌情考虑。

（二）麻醉选择

硬膜外麻醉或静脉麻醉。

（三）手术时机

1. 无异常子宫出血的患者可考虑月经干净 3～7 天后手术。

2. 异常子宫出血，经量多、经期长者一般在月经第 8 天后即可考虑手术。

3. 第一次手术没有切除干净，按照计划进行第二次宫腔镜手术切除者，一般第二次手术间隔时间在 1 个月后。

（四）术前准备

需行宫颈准备，根据患者具体情况可酌情选择以下方式中的一项：

1. 术前一晚宫颈备管。

2. 术前放置宫颈扩张棒扩张宫颈。

3. 术前阴道上药［米索前列醇 0.4 mg 或卡孕栓 1 mg（排除米索前列醇禁忌证）］软化宫颈，1 天 2 次，共 1～2 天。

4. 手术开始前 10 分钟静脉给予间苯三酚软化宫颈。

（五）术前评估

对子宫肌瘤进行恰当的分类对于指导治疗方案选择，包括手术方案选择都具有重要意义。推荐使用 STEP-W 子宫黏膜下肌瘤分类系统来预测复杂手术、肌瘤切除不完整、手术时间长、液体超载和其他主要并发症的发生（推荐等级 1B）。Ricardo Lasmar 提出的 STEP-W 分类，基于对五个子宫黏膜下肌瘤特征进行打分：大小、形态、基底延伸、穿透范围和侧壁位置（表 2-1）。前瞻性多中心研究表明，与欧洲妇科内镜学会（European Society for Gastrointestinal Endoscopy，ESGE）先前提出的分类系统相比，STEP-W 分类可以更好地预测复杂宫腔镜下子宫肌瘤去除术（hysteroscopic myomectomy，HM）的手术时间、肌瘤切除是否完整、液体平衡、并发症的发生率和严重程度。由于 HM 可能需要两次或更多次手术才可完成，STEP-W 评分系统能够比仅基于子宫肌瘤大小和肌壁穿透程度的评分系统更好地预测两次或更多次手术的风险。

表 2-1　黏膜下肌瘤的 STEP-W 分类

分数	大小	形态	基底延伸	穿透范围	侧壁位置
0	<2 cm	低	<1/3	0	+1
1	2～5 cm	中	1/3～2/3	<50%	

续表

分数	大小	形态	基底延伸	穿透范围	侧壁位置
2	>5 cm	高	>2/3	>50%	
得分					
0~4	第一组	低复杂度 HM			
5~6	第二组	高复杂度 HM，分次 HM，GnRH-α 使用			
7~9	第三组	考虑替代 HM			

注：GnRH-α，促性腺激素释放激素；HM，宫腔镜下子宫肌瘤去除术。

（六）手术操作流程

1. 宫腔镜电切术：常规外阴、阴道消毒，宫颈扩张至 10~12 号。经宫颈置入宫腔电切镜，进行 HM 手术操作。

（1）0 型肌瘤（有蒂肌瘤）：

1）肌瘤体积不大时，宫腔镜下看准肌瘤之根蒂部，直接切断瘤蒂，以卵圆钳夹出瘤体。

2）肌瘤体积较大不能直接钳夹出来时，在宫腔内分次切割瘤体，使之体积缩小后再切断瘤蒂，卵圆钳夹出组织，切割肌瘤根蒂部时应距离肌瘤附着处 3~5 mm，避免周围内膜及肌层损伤。

3）对于脱入阴道的子宫颈部肌瘤，电切环自瘤蒂部切除瘤体或用卵圆抓钳将瘤体钳夹拧除后，再用宫腔镜环形电极切除瘤蒂。

（2）Ⅰ~Ⅱ型黏膜下肌瘤（无蒂肌瘤）：

1）通过宫腔电切镜针状电极或者环状电极在肌瘤表面切开覆盖在肌瘤的包膜，并用电剪或针状电极（不带电），适当分离肌瘤与包膜，切割窗不要太大，一般先以凸向宫腔部分的肌瘤直径大小为宜。然后降低膨宫压力，宫颈注射宫缩剂（缩宫素 10 U、麦角新碱 0.2 mg 或稀释的垂体后叶素 4 U）促进子宫收缩，使肌壁间肌瘤向宫腔内凸出更加明显，使肌瘤与包膜分离，更有利于手术将肌瘤完全切除干净。

2）用环状电极在包膜内电切肌瘤，上下或左右交替切割，使瘤体形成"沟槽"样结构；肌瘤和包膜一般有明显的分界，肌瘤呈灰白色，无血管，质地硬，包膜呈粉红色，表面血管丰富，可用电切镜的头端或者环状电极机械性地推动瘤体来识别肌瘤和包膜的分界。

3）当瘤体不断缩小，部分瘤体呈片状或者条状时，以卵圆抓钳钳夹部分瘤体，并向一个方向扭转，直至残余瘤体与子宫肌层完全剥离，然后可以再次切割，多次反复，按照"夏氏五步法"切割—钳夹—扭转—牵拉—娩出，最后完全切除肌瘤取出瘤体。并全面探查宫腔瘤体是否切除干净，有无活动性出血。

4）术中瘤床包膜表面有出血，可用环状电极电凝止血，并可再次加用宫缩剂促进子宫收缩止血。

（3）Ⅲ型肌壁间肌瘤：该类肌瘤不属于黏膜下肌瘤，但由于肌瘤瘤体紧贴于黏膜下，可能稍凸或者不凸向子宫腔，Ⅲ型肌壁间肌瘤的根蒂埋藏在子宫肌层，瘤体表面有被覆黏膜层及子宫肌层组织，术前需结合影像学及术者经验充分评估。手术中应先行划开肌瘤表面被覆的黏膜层与肌层，待肌瘤凸向子宫腔内，然后按Ⅱ型黏膜下肌瘤处理，操作方法同无蒂黏膜下肌瘤。如若切开肌瘤表面被覆内膜后肌瘤不向子宫腔内凸入，应停止手术操作，在瘤体表面开窗后，肌壁间的瘤体可能随着子宫收缩慢慢凸向宫腔，根据其大小和有无临床症状，选择适当的方法切除肌瘤。手术必须在全程超声监测下进行。

2. 机械性旋转切除术：

（1）0型肌瘤（有蒂肌瘤）：将机械性组织切除装置的操作窗直接紧贴瘤体表面，在瘤体表面旋切，逐渐旋切瘤体使之体积缩小后再旋切瘤蒂，以免先旋瘤蒂后瘤体在宫腔内漂浮，组织切除装置无法紧贴瘤体。同时应该注意的是旋切根蒂部时应距离肌瘤附着处 3～5 mm，避免周围内膜及肌层损伤。

（2）Ⅰ型黏膜下肌瘤（无蒂肌瘤）：将机械性组织切除装置的操作窗直接紧贴瘤体表面，在瘤体表面旋切，逐渐旋切瘤体使之体积缩小，当旋切到肌层内的瘤体时，酌情给予缩宫素促使子宫收缩，使生长在子宫肌壁间的肌瘤组织突向子宫腔，便于通过切割窗旋切；如瘤体与包膜之间可见间隙，也可用切除装置的头端将瘤体与肌层的包膜轻轻分离，于瘤体与包膜的间隙内放置组织切除装置，注意要在直视下确认肌瘤组织，将切割窗紧贴肌瘤，逐渐旋切全部包膜内的肌瘤组织。

（七）术中术后注意事项

1. 术中肌瘤基底较宽，切除肌壁内肌瘤组织时必须识别肌瘤包膜与子宫肌壁的分界，肌瘤为不含血管的灰白色致密组织，而子宫宫壁是粉红色网格状且富含血管的组织。一定要在直视下确认肌瘤组织，最好通过各种方法使肌瘤向宫腔凸出后再电切，切忌通过作用电极向子宫肌壁深处"掏挖"肌瘤，以免盲目电切导致子宫穿孔及周围脏器的电损伤。

2. 应注重保护子宫内膜，术中切开肌瘤的包膜时最好选用电剪或针状电极，如果选用环状电极切开包膜，切割窗不宜过大，术中应该尽量保留肌瘤表面的包膜，以利于手术后包膜覆盖瘤床，避免术中宫腔粘连的发生。对于前后壁"对吻"位置的多发性肌瘤，一般分次手术，以免术后对吻面宫腔粘连。用机械性宫腔组织切除系统时，切割窗需要距离肌瘤附着处 3~5 mm，避免周围内膜及肌层损伤，避免手术创面宫腔粘连。黏膜下肌瘤术后对于有生育要求者建议采用预防宫腔粘连的措施，研究表明交联透明质酸钠治疗的患者术后粘连发生率与未接受治疗组相比降低。

3. HM 手术应在超声监护下实施，对于较大肌瘤的宫腔镜手术，通过超声监导能够提示宫腔镜切割电极作用的方向和深度，肌层的厚度，提示并能够及时发现子宫穿孔。

4. 术中是否需要腹腔镜监护，应根据具体情况而定。对于较大的黏膜下肌瘤，特别是肌瘤表面浆肌层厚度<0.5 cm 的患者，在腹腔镜监护下实施手术则更为安全，腹腔镜直视下能够协助判断肌瘤经宫腔镜切除的可行性，如宫腔镜无法完成时，可经腹腔镜剔除肌瘤；与此同时，能够及时发现不全子宫穿孔，进行穿孔修补及其他相应处理。

5. 宫腔镜手术切除较大、较多或位置较深的肌瘤时，术中和术后可有较多量的出血。术中出血较多时可提高灌流液压力，应用血管收缩药物，宫腔镜电极电凝等方法止血。对于肌瘤切除手术结束时的较多量出血，可考虑应用球囊导管压迫导尿管止血。宫腔 Foley 球囊压迫止血的操作方法如下：①先于导管球囊内注入 1~3 mL 气体作为球囊边缘指示，用剪刀剪去球囊顶端的导管。注意不要剪破球囊。②手术结束时行 B 超引导，将 Foley 导尿管植入宫腔，向球囊内注入适量无菌生理盐水，同时观察阴道出血情况。③导尿管末端收集袋，收集并观察宫腔内出血情况。④根据患者的宫腔大小和子宫肌瘤大小，球囊注水量一般为 10~30 mL，并且球囊内的液体注入量应少于切除标本量；B 超所见球囊大小应小于术前肌瘤的大小。⑤一般球囊宫腔内压迫防治时间为 6~8 小时。可一次取出，也可分次抽液减压再取出。在球囊留置期间如出血量增多，可再向球囊内加注液体，压迫止血。

6. 对于大的肌瘤，手术时间尽量控制在 1 小时以内，育龄期的健康女性在使用双极进行以生理盐水为膨宫介质的宫腔镜下子宫肌瘤去除术中，液体负欠量小于 1 000 mL 时，主要并发症的发生风险较低。液体负欠量 1 000~2 500 mL 时需要进行严密监测，在出现可能发生栓塞的细微征象时停止手术。液体负欠量超过 2 500 mL 时需要立即终止手术（推荐等级 1C 级）。对于老年人以及患有心血管、肾脏或其他合并症的女性，液体负欠量阈值应降低至 750 mL（推荐等级 1B 级）。手术时间超过半小时，即可用呋塞米 20 mg 减少体内容量负荷，如果手术时间超过 1 小时，肌瘤未切除干净者，可采用分次手术。术后如需要宫腔内留置球囊压迫止血，球囊留置时间不宜太长，以免引起宫内感染。少量残留在深肌层的肌瘤组织日后可能坏死吸收，对于不能吸收的肌瘤，如术后复查超声如果瘤体位于肌壁间未向宫腔内突出，可定期随访月经情况及肌瘤大小，如超声提示向宫腔内突出，可进行二次手术，第二次手术一般安排在至少 1 个月后。

（八）诊治流程（图 2-1）

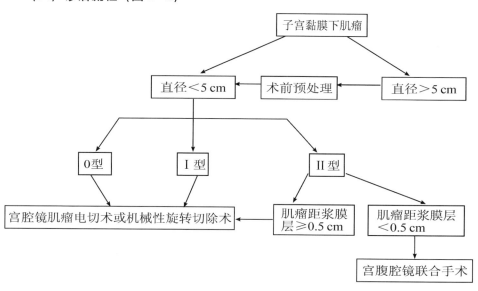

图 2-1　子宫黏膜下肌瘤诊治流程

周静　刘秋红

【参考文献】

[1] 子宫肌瘤诊治中国专家共识专家组. 子宫肌瘤诊治中国专家共识 [J].

中华妇产科杂志，2017，52（12）：793−800.

　　[2] 王艳霞，孟跃进，廖予妹，等. 宫腔镜下子宫黏膜下肌瘤电切术并发症的防治 [J]. 江苏医药，2013，39（11）：1317−1319.

　　[3] 汪静. 宫腔镜治疗子宫黏膜下肌瘤疗效研究 [J]. 实用妇科内分泌杂志（电子版），2016，3（4）：119−121.

　　[4] 段华. 子宫黏膜下肌瘤的宫腔镜治疗 [J]. 中国实用妇科与产科杂志，2016，32（2）：123−126.

　　[5] 王晓雷，李文学，臧红霞，等. 宫腔镜电切术治疗Ⅱ型子宫黏膜下肌瘤两种切除方法对生殖预后的影响 [J]. 中国实用妇科与产科杂志，2017，33（4）：423−427.

　　[6] 陈丽梅，张宏伟，谢侇，等. FIGO 3 型子宫肌瘤经宫腔镜电切手术的临床探索研究 [J]. 中华妇产科杂志，2022，57（10）：746−752.

　　[7] 王美藏，邓姗. 3 型子宫肌瘤的临床意义 [J]. 生殖医学杂志，2022，31（1）：94−97.

　　[8] 黄东静. 肌壁间子宫肌瘤宫腔镜切除术的可行性及患者生殖预后研究 [J]. 中国医疗器械信息，2020，26（22）：39−40.

　　[9] 黄睿，黄晓武，夏恩兰，等. 宫腔镜下 3 型子宫肌瘤切除术可行性及生殖预后分析 [J]. 国际生殖健康/计划生育杂志，2018，37（1）：24−28.

　　[10] 褚春芳，吴玉梅. 无宫腔受压肌壁间子宫肌瘤对妊娠影响的研究进展 [J]. 中国医药导报，2019，16（24）：47−50.

　　[11] Alessandro Loddo, Dusan Djokovic, Amal Driz, et al. Hysteroscopic myomectomy: the guidelines of the International Society for Gynecologic Endoscopy (ISGE) [J]. Eur J Obstet Gynecol Reprod Biol, 2022, 268: 121−128.

　　[12] MAIS V, CIRRONIS M G, PEIRETTI M, et al. Efficacy of autocrosslinked hyaluronan gel for adhesion prevention in laparoscopy and hysteroscopy: a systematic review and meta-analysis of randomized controlled trials [J]. Eur J Obstet Gynecol Reprod Biol, 2012, 160 (1): 1−5.

　　[13] CHENG M, CHANG W H, YANG S T, et al. Efficacy of applying hyaluronic acid gels in the primary prevention of intrauterine adhesion after hysteroscopic myomectomy: a meta-analysis of randomized controlled trials [J]. Life (Basel), 2020, 10 (11): 285.

第三章　剖宫产切口部妊娠
诊治流程及手术操作规范

剖宫产切口部妊娠（cesarean scar pregnancy，CSP）是指受精卵着床于前次剖宫产子宫切口瘢痕处的一种异位妊娠，是一个限时定义，仅限于妊娠早期（≤12 周）。CSP 的发生率为 1∶2 216～1∶1 800，占有前次剖宫产史妇女的1.15%，占有前次剖宫产史妇女异位妊娠的 6.1%。由于 CSP 可以造成清宫手术中及术后难以控制的大出血、子宫破裂、周围器官损伤，甚至切除子宫等，严重威胁妇女的生殖健康甚至生命，已引起临床上的高度重视。

一、诊断

1. 临床表现：有停经史，阴道少量流血，轻微下腹痛等先兆流产的表现。

2. 体格检查：妇科检查表现为子宫增大、质软等妊娠子宫体征。

3. 辅助检查：

（1）超声表现：①宫腔内、子宫颈管内空虚，未见妊娠囊；②妊娠囊着床于子宫前壁下段肌层（相当于前次剖宫产子宫切口部位），部分妊娠囊内可见胎芽或胎心搏动；③子宫前壁肌层连续性中断，妊娠囊与膀胱之间的子宫肌层明显变薄，甚至消失；③彩色多普勒血流成像（color Doppler flow imaging，CDFI）显示妊娠囊周边高速低阻血流信号。

（2）磁共振成像：磁共振成像（magnetic resonance imaging，MRI）检查矢状面及横断面的 T_1、T_2 加权连续扫描均能清晰地显示子宫前壁下段内的妊娠囊与子宫及其周围器官的关系。

（3）血清人绒毛膜促性腺激素：呈阳性，对于异常升高的人绒毛膜促性腺激

素 β 亚单位（human chorionic gonadotropin-β，β-HCG）也要警惕是否合并妊娠滋养细胞肿瘤。β-HCG 在治疗后的随诊中评价治疗效果时非常重要。

二、分型

2016 年，《剖宫产术后子宫瘢痕妊娠诊治专家共识》根据超声检查显示的着床于子宫前壁瘢痕处的妊娠囊的生长方向，以及子宫前壁妊娠囊与膀胱间子宫肌层的厚度进行分型，此分型方法有利于临床的实际操作。

Ⅰ型：①妊娠囊部分着床于子宫瘢痕处，部分或大部分位于宫腔内，少数甚或达宫底部宫腔；②妊娠囊明显变形、拉长，下端呈锐角；③妊娠囊与膀胱间子宫肌层变薄，厚度>3 mm；④CDFI：瘢痕处见滋养层血流信号（低阻血流）。

Ⅱ型：①妊娠囊部分着床于子宫瘢痕处，部分或大部分位于宫腔内，少数甚或达宫底部宫腔；②妊娠囊明显变形、拉长，下端呈锐角；③妊娠囊与膀胱间子宫肌层变薄，厚度≤3 mm；④CDFI：瘢痕处见滋养层血流信号（低阻血流）。

Ⅲ型：①妊娠囊完全着床于子宫瘢痕处肌层并向膀胱方向外凸；②宫腔及子宫颈管内空虚；③妊娠囊与膀胱之间子宫肌层明显变薄，甚或缺失，厚度≤3 mm；④CDFI：瘢痕处见滋养层血流信号（低阻血流）。

其中，Ⅲ型中还有 1 种特殊的超声表现 CSP，即包块型，其声像图的特点：①位于子宫下段瘢痕处的混合回声（呈囊实性）包块，有时呈类实性，包块向膀胱方向隆起；②包块与膀胱间子宫肌层明显变薄，甚或缺失；③CDFI：包块周边见较丰富的血流信号，可为低阻血流，少数也可仅见少许血流信号或无血流信号。包块型多见于 CSP 流产后（如药物流产后或负压吸引术后）子宫瘢痕处妊娠物残留并出血所致。

张洪文教授提出根据患者风险情况，进行分类后决定处理时机；根据子宫切口肌壁最薄处厚度，进行分型确定处理方式；根据病灶位置高低，分亚型选择手术路径，具体如下：

第一步分类，根据患者风险情况，决定处理时机。根据就诊时是否有大出血风险，分为风险型 CSP 和稳定型 CSP。风险型 CSP 一般有如下特征之一：①曾有或正在自发出血；②宫腔操作中（如人工流产时）发生出血；②B 超提示病灶心管搏动明显；③血 β-HCG 较高，提示绒毛活性强。这类患者需尽快做出决定降低其大出血的风险。稳定型 CSP 的血 β-HCG 不高或正常，影像学或 B 超未见心管搏动，其具有极低的出血风险，其病情稳定，几乎无出血风险，可以择期手术治疗。

第二步分型，根据子宫切口肌壁最薄处厚度，确定处理方式。风险型 CSP 又可以根据原切口部位子宫壁最薄处厚薄程度（以 3 mm 为界）分为壁薄型 CSP 和壁厚型 CSP。壁薄型 CSP 局部子宫壁较薄，不能承受吸刮时的冲击力，选择外科手术切开子宫瘢痕处并清除局部病灶，再行切口部位修补术。壁厚型（Ⅱ型）CSP（局部子宫壁最薄处厚度≥3 mm）则选择吸刮术处理。

第三步分亚型，根据病灶位置高低，选择手术路径。根据剖宫产时切口位置的高低以及局部包块的大小将壁薄型 CSP 分为位置较低型（Ⅰa 型）CSP、位置较高型（Ⅰb 型）CSP 和外凸巨块型（Ⅰc 型）CSP（包块直径>5 cm），用以辅助选择具体手术路径。位置的确定目前仍需要结合妇科检查判断，位置较低型 CSP 建议选择经阴道入路手术清除病灶，可以减少手术操作的难度，而位置较高型及外凸巨块型建议选择开腹手术或腹腔镜手术清除病灶则难度会小一些。具体术式的选择也需要结合患者情况、手术医师熟练程度以及当地治疗水平及条件综合确定。风险型 CSP 若胚胎组织只有一部分位于剖宫产切口部位（<50%），则称之为偏移型（Ⅲ型）CSP，同样也适合吸刮术来解决，此类型需要与宫内正常妊娠区分，尽管病灶部分位于切口部位，但也有一定的大出血风险，故对此类 CSP 需积极处理，在临床上进一步引起重视。稳定型 CSP 虽然没有大出血风险，但一般清宫吸宫治疗很难将其彻底解决，建议行宫腔镜电切术。CSP 临床分型及优化治疗流程图见图 3-1。

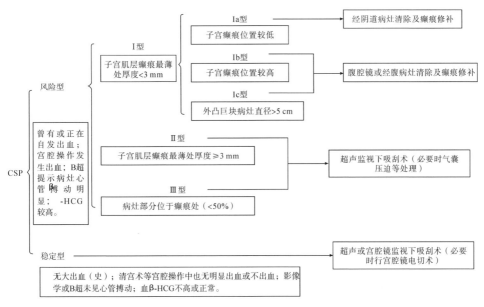

图 3-1　张洪文教授 CSP 临床分型及优化治疗流程图

山东大学齐鲁医院根据多年临床经验总结的实用临床分型。根据经阴道多普勒超声（transvaginal Doppler，TVD）诊断将瘢痕妊娠分为 3 型（表3-1）。

表 3-1　齐鲁医院 CSP 实用临床分型

实用临床分型	最小前壁肌层厚度	包块或妊娠囊平均直径	推荐的首选手术方式
Ⅰ	>3 mm	无论大小	超声监视下吸宫术＋宫腔镜手术*
Ⅱ	≤3 mm，且>1 mm	≤3 cm	超声监视下吸宫术＋宫腔镜手术*
		>3 cm	腹腔镜监视下吸宫术＋宫腔镜手术*或经阴道前穹窿切开病灶清除术 必要时瘢痕缺陷修补术
Ⅲ	≤1 mm	≤6 cm	腹腔镜下瘢痕妊娠病灶清除术＋吸宫术或经阴道前穹窿切开病灶清除术
		>6 cm，或伴有动静脉瘘	开腹手术或子宫动脉栓塞后腹腔镜手术

* 宫腔镜主要用于判断病灶是否清除干净，若有病灶残留可行宫腔镜残留病灶电切术。

三、鉴别诊断

1. 子宫颈妊娠：为妊娠囊着床于子宫颈管内，但子宫前壁下段的肌层连续性无中断。盆腔检查时，可发现子宫颈膨大，甚至可呈上小下大的葫芦形，子宫颈可呈紫蓝色，但子宫颈外口闭合。鉴别时主要依据是否有剖宫产史，超声检查妊娠囊着床的位置能进一步明确诊断。当妊娠周数较大或包块较大时，区分起来可能比较困难，如患者有剖宫产史，应高度怀疑 CSP。

2. 宫内妊娠难免流产：当宫内妊娠难免流产时，宫内妊娠囊向体外排出时暂时停留于前次剖宫产子宫瘢痕处，此时超声检查可以在子宫瘢痕部位见妊娠囊或混合回声包块。鉴别时要注意病史，如有腹痛、阴道流血、子宫颈口张开，多是宫内早孕，难免流产。此外，超声检查需注意妊娠囊或包块在子宫瘢痕处有无高速低阻血流，前次剖宫产子宫瘢痕处的肌层是否有连续性中断。

3. 妊娠滋养细胞肿瘤：CSP 清宫不全或不全流产后残留的妊娠物继续生长在子宫前壁下段形成包块，其超声影像类似于妊娠滋养细胞肿瘤的表现，如与肌层无明显界线、局部肌层缺如或变薄、局部血流信号极其丰富、可探及高速低阻血流，甚至出现动静脉瘘的花色血流信号等，易误诊为妊娠滋养细胞肿瘤。但 CSP 有明确的剖宫产史，常常有人工流产或药物流产史，包块位于子宫前壁下段，与子宫瘢痕关系密切，且血 β-HCG 水平通常不会很高，很少超过 100 000 U/L。结合病史和辅助检查应首先考虑 CSP 的可能，不要盲目按照妊娠滋养细胞肿瘤进行化疗。

四、治疗

（一）手术指征

CSP 作为一种特殊类型的异位妊娠，诊治原则是早诊断，早终止，早清除。早诊断是指对有剖宫产史的妇女再次妊娠时应尽早行超声检查排除 CSP。一旦诊断为 CSP 应给出终止妊娠的医学建议，并尽早清除妊娠物。如患者因自身原因坚决要求继续妊娠，应交待继续妊娠可能发生的风险和并发症，如前置胎盘、胎盘植入、子宫破裂等所致的产时或产后难以控制的大出血，甚至子宫切除、危及生命等险恶结局。

（二）麻醉选择

静脉麻醉或者硬膜外椎管内麻醉。

（三）手术时机选择

剖宫产切口部妊娠诊断明确后尽早手术。

（四）手术前预处理

1. 子宫动脉栓塞术（uterine arterial embolization，UAE）：

适应证：①用于 CSP 终止妊娠的手术时或自然流产时发生大出血需要紧急止血的情况；②Ⅱ型和Ⅲ型 CSP，包块型血液供应丰富者，手术前预处理行子宫动脉栓塞术，以减少清宫手术或 CSP 妊娠物清除手术中的出血风险，因介入治疗后可导致宫腔粘连、卵巢功能减退的并发症，主要适用于无生育要求的患者。

2. 高强度聚焦超声（high intensity focused ultrasound，HIFU）：

适应证：①孕周≤10 周，孕囊径线≤40 mm 的 CSP 患者；②机载超声可显示病灶，位于超声路径，焦域可容纳，有安全声通道及有效焦距；③依据超声检查显示的着床于子宫前壁瘢痕处的妊娠囊的生长方向，以及子宫前壁妊娠囊与膀胱间子宫肌层型为Ⅰ型、Ⅱ型的患者；④自愿接受镇静镇痛下超声消融治疗并签署同意书。治疗主要针对孕囊及周边组织，不影响卵巢及子宫内膜功能，故主要适用于有生育要求的患者。

（五）手术操作规范

1. 超声监测下宫腔镜清宫术：

（1）手术适应证：患者生命体征平稳，孕周<8 周的Ⅰ型 CSP。Ⅱ型、Ⅲ型 CSP 及孕周>8 周的Ⅰ型 CSP 宫腔镜下清宫术前需进行预处理。宫腔镜下胚物去除是 TURP 和空气栓塞的高风险手术，围手术期必须做好防范措施。

（2）宫腔镜手术操作流程：

1）患者取膀胱截石位，静脉麻醉，常规消毒手术部位，膨宫液采用生理盐水，行宫腔检查镜确定病灶部位。

2）先吸子宫中上段及下段后壁的蜕膜组织，再尽量吸取子宫下段的妊娠囊，之后以较小的压力［200～300 mmHg（26.7～40.0 kPa）］清理剖宫产瘢痕部位的蜕膜及残留的绒毛组织。

3）再次置入宫腔镜检查宫腔情况，对残留组织予微型钳钳夹去除或予宫腔镜电切去除残留组织，如瘢痕部位有粘连带，先剪开瘢痕部位的粘连带，再将粘连带后方的妊娠物清除。

4）如妊娠物位于切口下缘活瓣的后方，则考虑用环状电极机械性刮除。如为机化妊娠残留组织,刮除困难,可用环状电极切除切口下缘活瓣后电切妊娠残留物。

5)出血较多时可宫腔镜电凝止血或宫腔填塞水囊压迫止血。在超声指引下将水囊置入剖宫产瘢痕妊娠部位,囊内注入生理盐水,超声下见水囊与切口妊娠部位肌层紧贴,即停止注水,然后接引流袋,观察引流袋内有无血液活动性流出,如仍有出血,可再向囊内注入生理盐水,一般注入 10~50 mL 均能压迫止血。

6)水囊管一般24~48 小时取出,放出囊内液体前先注射缩宫剂,可分两次或者一次放出囊内液体。一般囊内注水超过 30 mL,分两次放出囊内液体更安全。

2. 宫腔镜联合腹腔镜手术操作规范:

(1)手术适应证:Ⅱ型和Ⅲ型 CSP,特别是Ⅲ型中的包块型,子宫前壁瘢痕处肌层菲薄,血流丰富,有再生育要求并希望同时修补子宫缺损,特别是剖宫产瘢痕位置高,子宫前壁与前腹壁粘连的患者。

(2)手术操作流程及注意事项:

1)患者取膀胱截石位,气管插管全身麻醉,先宫腔镜检查,明确病灶部位,再行腹腔镜手术。

2)予举宫器举宫,腹腔镜下用超声刀打开膀胱子宫返折腹膜,下推膀胱逐渐至病灶下方,以便有足够的空间切除病灶。

3)切开子宫肌层,切除病灶及其周边瘢痕组织,用 2-0 可吸收线间断缝合切口,注意切口部位缝合要对齐,特别是两侧角部,以免切口愈合后再次形成憩室。

4)再次置入宫腔镜检查宫腔是否有病灶残留及切口缝合情况。切除物常规送病理检查。也可以先行腹腔镜探查子宫大小、形态,子宫前峡部瘢痕处隆突程度,妊娠包块大小、表面颜色,是否盆腔粘连等。根据探查结果先在宫腔镜检查及腹腔镜监护下行负压吸宫术,大部分妊娠物清除后可行腹腔镜下瘢痕缺陷修补术。

3. 经阴道病灶切除手术操作规范:

(1)手术适应证:Ⅱ型和Ⅲ型 CSP,妊娠<10 周或包块直径<6 cm,子宫前壁瘢痕处肌层菲薄,血流丰富,有再生育要求并希望同时修补子宫缺损的患者,

特别是剖官产瘢痕位置低，子官前壁与前腹壁无粘连的患者。

（2）手术操作流程及注意事项：

1）患者取膀胱截石位，腰硬联合麻醉或气管插管全身麻醉，于官颈、阴道交界处膀胱沟水平，注入生理盐水形成水垫。沿膀胱沟水平横行切开阴道壁，组织剪沿官颈撑开膀胱官颈间隙，用两个巾钳向下牵拉官颈，用食指向上方及双侧钝性上推膀胱。如果粘连紧密也可锐性分离，至膀胱腹膜返折处，可不打开返折腹膜，但要有足够的空间切除病灶组织。

2）见到病灶组织后，切开子官至官腔，用组织钳钳夹切缘，切除病灶及周边瘢痕组织，清除官内蜕膜组织。

3）用2-0可吸收线间断缝合切口全层，先不打结，预留打结线头长度，弯钳钳夹线头，缝合完毕分别打结，检查推开的膀胱创面无活动性出血点，再连续缝合前穹隆阴道壁。

4）行官腔镜检查，再次检查官腔内是否有残留组织及缝合处情况。切除物常规送病理检查。

（六）围手术期注意事项

1. 术前充分评估术中出血的风险，可行预防性的子官动脉栓塞术或 HIFU 减少术中出血。

2. 官腹腔镜联合的患者可术中行子官动脉临时阻断，减少术中出血。

3. 术中注意加强官缩，术中当孕囊吸出后可用缩官素 10 U 官颈注射，如果术中官缩欠佳可加用麦角新碱 0.2 mg 官颈注射，或者垂体后叶素 3~6 U 官颈注射，或者肛门内上卡孕栓 1 mg 或米索前列醇 0.4 mg。

4. 官腹腔镜和经阴道病灶切除术的患者交代术中出血多时，必要时需要中转开腹手术，无法控制的大出血必要时需要切除子官。

（七）诊治流程（图 3-2）

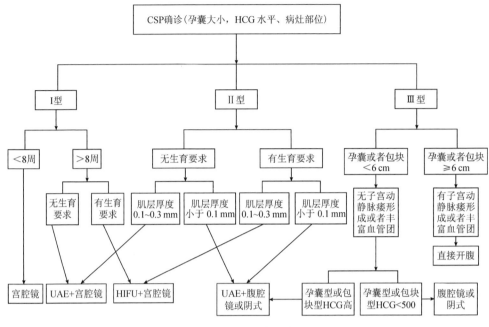

图 3-2　CSP 诊治流程

刘秋红

【参考文献】

［1］中华医学会妇产科学医学分会计划生育组. 剖宫产术后子宫瘢痕妊娠诊治专家共识［J］. 中华妇产科杂志，2016，51（8）：568-571.

［2］陈春林. 剖宫产瘢痕部位妊娠诊治进展［J］. 实用妇产科杂志，2017，33（4）：245-248.

［3］左娜，张宁宁. 宫腔镜手术对于不同临床分型早孕期剖宫产瘢痕妊娠的治疗效果分析［J］. 生殖医学杂志，2018，27（5）：395-398.

［4］段华，孙馥箐. 内镜在剖宫产瘢痕妊娠诊治中的应用［J］. 实用妇产科杂志，2014，30（4）：249-25.

［5］张洪文. 剖宫产术后瘢痕处妊娠的临床分型、优化治疗及其意义［J］. 国际妇产科学杂志，2017，44（3）：315-318.

［6］袁岩，戴晴，蔡胜，等. 超声在剖宫产瘢痕妊娠诊断的诊断价值［J］. 中华超声影像学杂志，2010，19（4）：321-324.

［7］LIU S，SUN J，CAI B，et al. Management of Cesarean Scar Pregnancy Using Ultrasound-Guided Dilation and Curettage ［J］. J Minim Invasive Gynecol，2016，23（5）：707－711.

［8］康彦君，班艳丽，张腾，等. 子宫瘢痕妊娠实用临床分型及应用价值探讨 ［J］. 现代妇产科进展，2019，28（10）：731－735.

［9］陈芳，臧春逸. 高强度聚焦超声在剖宫产瘢痕妊娠中的应用 ［J］. 医学影像学杂志，2021，31（1）：110－112，118.

［10］XIAO J H，ZHANG S H，WANG F，et al. Cesarean scar pregnancy：noninvasive andeffective treatment with high-intensity focused ultrasound ［J］. Am J Obstet Gynecol，2014，211（4）：356－363.

［11］ZHANG Y，ZHANG C，HE J，et al. The impact of gestational sac size on the effectiveness and safety of high intensity focused ultrasound combined with ultrasound-guided suction curettage treatment for caesarean scar pregnancy ［J］. Int J Hyperthermia，2018，35（1）：291－297.

第四章　剖宫产切口憩室
诊治流程及手术操作规范

剖宫产切口憩室（cesarean scar diverticulum，CSD）又称为剖宫产子宫切口缺损（previous cesarean scar defect，PCSD），指剖宫产术后子宫切口愈合不良，子宫瘢痕处肌层变薄，形成一道与宫腔相通的凹陷或腔隙，导致部分患者出现一系列相关的临床症状。CSD作为剖宫产术的远期并发症，发生率为$19.4\%\sim88.0\%$，并且随着检查手段及对疾病认识的提高，临床的实际发生率更高，该病可对患者的生命质量造成影响，且再次妊娠时可增加剖宫产切口部妊娠（cesarean scar pregnancy，CSP）、大出血、凶险性前置胎盘、子宫破裂等的风险。

一、诊断

1. 临床表现：

（1）有子宫下段剖宫产手术史。

（2）有以异常阴道流血为主的临床症状：经期延长、经间期出血、性交后流血、不孕等（异常阴道流血多数出现在剖宫产术半年后）。其他有痛经、盆腔痛、子宫瘢痕撕裂，以及瘢痕子宫妊娠等。

2. 体格检查：妇科检查子宫双附件多无异常。

3. 辅助检查：

（1）三维经阴道超声（three-dimension transvaginal ultrasound，3D-TVS）：最简便、最常用的检查方法，但敏感度及特异度均不高，最佳检查时机需在有临床症状时，即经期或阴道不规则流血时。典型的超声影像学表现为子宫前壁下段剖宫产术后子宫切口处浆膜层连续而肌层不连续，存在1个或数个边缘模糊的楔形或囊状液性暗区,尖端突向浆膜面且与宫腔相通,此处子宫肌层厚度减小。

(2) 子宫输卵管造影(hysteron salpingography,HSG):表现为子宫下段的囊状结构或呈线状、带状缺损。检查时需向宫腔内加压注入造影剂,目前已逐渐被宫腔声学造影所取代。

(4) 宫腔声学造影(sonohysterography,SHG):将超声造影剂注入宫腔,经阴道行超声检查,待子宫前后壁内膜充分分离,见典型的子宫下段楔形或囊状液性暗区;同时观察宫腔内是否有占位性病变。由于造影剂增加了病变与宫壁之间的对比度,诊断的特异度及敏感度与 3D-TVS 相比均较高,尤其是对于无症状的 CSD 患者也有良好的诊断作用。

(5) 磁共振成像(magnetic resonance imaging,MRI):其特征表现为子宫前壁下段可见瘢痕影,局部变薄,龛影与宫腔相通。CSD 信号表现为 T_1 加权成像(weighted imaging,WI)等信号或高信号、T_2WI 高信号,其矢状位龛影形态大致可分为浅凹陷、三角形、小囊形及囊袋形 4 种。MRI 扫描 T_2 序列子宫瘢痕处呈低信号,对应部位的局部子宫肌层变薄,宫腔面内陷。T_1WI 序列增强扫描显示成熟的子宫瘢痕供血少,不强化或轻度强化,憩室显示明显,与宫腔相通。MRI 检查在显示软组织方面更具优势,能从多个平面更好地观察子宫瘢痕部位和所有子宫肌层的中断情况,缺点是价格较为昂贵。

(6) 宫腔镜检查:宫腔镜下可见子宫峡部前壁剖宫产术后子宫切口处凹陷形成憩室结构,切口下缘的纤维组织形成"活瓣",凹陷内可见陈旧积血或黏液,憩室内局部血管增生、迂曲扩张,有时可见较薄的子宫内膜生长。因宫腔镜的直视性等优点被认为是诊断 CSD 的最佳方法。

二、分型及分度

1. 分型:CSD 的分型方法众多,但尚无针对不同分型进行个体化治疗的方案,因此,分型对于临床的指导意义欠佳。目前按形状可分为囊状憩室和细线状憩室缺损;按位置可分为宫腔下段、子宫颈峡部和子宫颈上段;按照大小可分为肌层缺损<80% 的龛影(niche)和肌层缺损≥80% 的切口裂开(dehiscence)。

2. 分级:目前,国内关于 CSD 尚没有相关的分级标准。Tower 等结合临床症状和憩室大小等将其分为 3 度:2~3 分为轻度,4~6 分为中度,7~9 分为重度。分级标准如表 4-1 所示。

表 4-1　剖宫产瘢痕部位愈合缺陷的分级标准

类别	项目标准描述	分数/分
残存子宫肌层厚度/mm	SIS>2.2	1
	SIS≤2.2	3
	3D-TVS>2.5	1
	3D-TVS≤2.5	3
残存子宫肌层百分比/%	>50	1
	20~50	2
	<20	3
子宫其他瘢痕个数/个	1	0
	>1	1
剖宫产次数/次	1	0
	>1	1
月经	正常	0
	异常	1

注：残存子宫肌层百分比＝残存子宫肌层厚度/周围正常子宫肌层厚度×100%；SIS，注入生理盐水 B 超。

三、鉴别诊断

1. 子宫黏膜下肌瘤或内膜息肉：有月经过多或不规则阴道流血，可行超声检查、宫腔镜检查以及诊断性刮宫以明确诊断。

2. 子宫内膜癌：主要表现为阴道流血或阴道排液，病灶累及宫颈可出现宫腔积脓、下腹疼痛等。早期妇科检查无异常，晚期可有子宫增大，合并宫腔积脓时可有明显压痛。超声提示宫腔内不均质区，或宫腔线消失，肌层内不均回声区。

四、治疗

目前，CSD 的治疗包括药物治疗及手术治疗。

（一）药物治疗

主要包括激素治疗和止血治疗。

1. 激素治疗：包括口服短效避孕药和放置左炔诺孕酮宫内缓释节育系统

（LNG-IUS）两种常用方法。前者用药期间月经期较前缩短，月经淋漓症状消失，少数患者治疗无效；部分患者因避孕药禁忌证者而不能选用，且易出现停药后症状反复，依从性差。后者因在宫腔内恒定地释放一定量的孕激素从而抑制子宫内膜增生，使患者异常子宫出血时间大大缩短，甚至达到闭经的效果，从而改善或消除原有的症状。但部分患者在放置 LNG-IUS 后仍有月经净后少量持续点滴出血或原症状无明显改善，因此，CSD 患者放置 LNG-IUS 后出现的异常子宫出血是否为 LNG-IUS 相关的副作用或仍由 CSD 所致，在临床判断上容易混淆，造成患者不便。

2. 止血治疗：妥塞敏（氨甲环酸片）作为临床常用止血药，在治疗 CSD 患者异常子宫出血时不建议单独使用，应与其他药物联合应用以达到更好的止血效果，但目前对于这类研究的报道较少，且多为短期内止血的治疗手段。

（二）手术治疗

1. 手术指征：诊断为 CSD 且有相应的临床症状，影响患者的生命质量，患者有治疗需求。

（1）宫腔镜手术：适用于子宫前壁下段肌层厚度≥3 mm 的 CSD 患者。考虑到宫腔镜手术中的热效应及子宫穿孔的风险，有学者提出单纯宫腔镜手术治疗前，应运用 MRI 进行术前评估，MRI 测量憩室距离子宫浆膜层＞2 mm 者可使用宫腔镜。也有学者认为残余肌壁厚度应选择在 2.5 mm 以上，Li 等则认为残余肌壁厚度应在 3.5 mm 以上。但目前行宫腔镜手术的指征（即残余肌层厚度）尚没有国际标准，据上述文献报道，憩室残余肌层厚度至少应大于 2 mm。

（2）宫腔镜联合腹腔镜：适用于子宫前壁下段肌层厚度＜3 mm 且有再生育要求的患者，特别是子宫腹壁有粘连的患者。也有学者提出对于瘢痕憩室处肌壁厚度小于 2.5 mm 者，可采用腹腔镜手术。

（3）阴式剖宫产子宫瘢痕憩室修补术：适用于子宫前壁下段肌层厚度＜3 mm 且有再生育要求的患者，特别是子宫腹壁无粘连的患者。也有学者提出对于瘢痕憩室处肌壁厚度小于 2.5 mm 者，可采用经阴道手术。该术式适用于有丰富阴道手术经验的医生操作，尤其适合于瘢痕憩室位置较低的患者。

2. 麻醉方式：①静脉全麻；②硬膜外或区域阻滞麻醉；③全身麻醉。

3. 手术时机：月经前半周期（9~13 天）。

4. 术前准备：

（1）病情告知与知情同意：根据患者病情选择合适的手术方式，但手术的疗效为 80%～95%，必要时术后需要辅助药物治疗，或者药物治疗症状也无明显改善。

（2）宫颈准备：根据患者具体情况可酌情选择不同方式。

1）术前晚宫颈备管。

2）术前放置宫颈扩张棒扩张宫颈。

3）术前阴道上药［米索前列醇 0.4 mg 或卡孕栓 1 mg（排除米索前列醇禁忌证）］软化宫颈。

4）手术开始前 10 分钟静脉给予间苯三酚软化宫颈。

（3）术前禁食 6～8 小时。

5. 手术操作规范：

（1）宫腔镜子宫瘢痕憩室矫治术手术操作规范：

1）患者取膀胱截石位，静脉麻醉，常规消毒外阴及阴道，用宫颈钳夹持宫颈前唇，扩张宫颈 10 号。

2）常规用生理盐水膨宫，膨宫压力 100～120 mmHg（13.3～16.0 kPa），先检查宫底、宫腔壁，再检查子宫角及输卵管开口，发现憩室部位，憩室内有无陈旧性积血、积脓，有无新生物及异常血管，切口下缘有无活瓣。

3）应用宫腔镜环状电极将 CSD 下缘凸起部分切除，一般先切除作双侧切口下缘的活瓣，最后切除紧靠膀胱下缘的活瓣，使整个切除处与假腔的内壁周围组织持平，使憩室内壁与内膜呈钝角，从而去除无效腔。

4）用球形电极电凝憩室部位增生的血管及内膜。注意电凝的功率和时间，避免膀胱电热损伤。

（2）宫腔镜联合腹腔镜子宫瘢痕憩室修补术手术操作规范：

1）患者取膀胱截石位，气管插管，全身麻醉。

2）先宫腔镜检查 CSD 部位、大小并进行透光试验。

3）换举宫器举宫，腹腔镜下用超声刀打开膀胱子宫反折腹膜，下推膀胱，如果盆腔有粘连可一并分离，下推膀胱时注意解剖层次不要伤及膀胱；如果没有把握，可用金属导尿管指引膀胱边缘，逐渐下推膀胱至 CSD 下方，以便有足够的空间切除 CSD 或者折叠缝合 CSD。

4）当采用手术切除 CSD 时，剪刀剪开憩室，切除瘢痕组织；用 2-0 可吸收线镜下间断缝合切口，注意切口两侧角的部位缝合要对齐，以免愈合后形成小的憩室，间断缝合5~6针；缝合时将简易举宫器的金属杆作为指引，每一针均不打结，预留出打结线的长度，间断缝合完毕，分别打结，再连续缝合切开的反折腹膜。

5）当采用手术折叠缝合CSD时，打开子宫膀胱反折腹膜，下推膀胱，形成新鲜创面后，可见子宫下段瘢痕薄弱处组织部分内陷，或选择宫腔镜透光明显处，沿肌层表面，采用聚对二氧环己酮（polydioxanone）材料制成的单向锚钩无菌1-0可吸收性单股缝线（也称鱼骨线），连续缝合憩室外壁上下端子宫下段肌层。缝合后，薄弱的肌层组织折叠加厚了下段肌层，缝合时需注意在缝合瘢痕两侧正常肌层时不要穿透宫腔，经宫腔镜再次探查憩室部位，此时憩室腔应平坦。腹腔镜下确认创面无活动性出血后，用可吸收缝线连续缝合膀胱子宫反折腹膜。

（3）阴式剖宫产子宫瘢痕憩室修补术手术操作规范：

1）患者取膀胱截石位，腰硬联合麻醉或气管插管全身麻醉。

2）于宫颈、阴道交界处膀胱沟水平，打水垫（可用生理盐水或者1∶20 000稀释的肾上腺素溶液）。

3）沿膀胱沟水平横行切开阴道壁达宫颈筋膜，薄剪沿宫颈撑开膀胱宫颈间隙。

4）用两个组织钳钳夹宫颈前后唇向下牵拉宫颈，用示指向上方及双侧钝性上推膀胱，如果粘连紧密也可锐性分离，至膀胱腹膜反折处，打开膀胱子宫腹膜反折，完全暴露憩室部位（可不打开反折腹膜，但要有足够的空间切除瘢痕组织）。

5）指腹于峡部压宫颈体交界处，CSD处触之稍有凹陷，用探针从宫颈外口进入宫颈管上分探查薄弱处，可扪及质地硬的探针，考虑此处为CSD，从此处切开瘢痕处至宫腔，有时可见暗红色黏液样物流出。

6）用组织钳钳夹切缘，切除薄弱处瘢痕组织，在扩宫条指引下用2-0可吸收线间断缝合切口全层，先不打结，预留打结线头长度，弯钳钳夹线头，缝合完毕，分别打结。

7）检查推开的膀胱创面无活动性出血点，再连续锁边或者连续缝合前穹隆阴道壁。

8）术毕行宫腔镜检查，检查宫腔形态，切口缝合部位有无憩室，退镜后阴道填塞络合碘纱布或纱条压迫阴道。

6. 术中术后注意事项：

（1）严格按照手术操作规程要求，实施无菌操作，动作轻柔，预防子宫及周围脏器损伤、感染、出血等并发症的发生；术后应使用抗生素预防感染，如有贫血或低蛋白血症，应及时对症处理，以尽量去除影响切口愈合的不良因素。

（2）宫腔镜手术时，建议术前用诊断性宫腔镜全面评估宫颈管，切口部位憩室大小，宫腔情况，了解宫腔走行，这样可以避免盲目探宫和扩张颈管时导致的子宫穿孔，手术操作时，假腔底部不能电切，只能用滚球电极电凝，且应注意电凝功率不宜过大，以免热损伤膀胱。用电切容易导致术中子宫穿孔，甚至膀胱损伤。术中一旦发现子宫穿孔，立即停止操作，并注射宫缩剂促进子宫收缩，根据是否合并膀胱损伤和穿孔处出血情况，以及是否有可能损伤其他脏器，而决定是否需要腹腔镜探查或者膀胱镜检查。

（3）宫腔镜电切手术时，憩室部位肌层薄，术中需要选择B超监护，同时需要稳定控制好电切镜，切除紧靠膀胱下缘的活瓣时切勿切入过深而误伤膀胱；切口假腔内膜只能用电凝，不能电切；尽量避免滚球电极在一个部位停留时间过长，以免电凝深度过深，导致膀胱热损伤。如果可疑膀胱损伤，需要请泌尿外科会诊，协助诊断和治疗。

（4）宫腔镜电切手术时，切除双侧切口下缘的活瓣时，切口太深而导致电切宫颈深度太深，可能损伤子宫动脉下行支，导致大出血。如出现子宫动脉损伤大出血，可通过在出血侧宫颈注射垂体后叶素后在宫腔镜直视下电凝出血的动脉，如果无效，可行子宫动脉栓塞术止血。

（5）经阴道手术术中应注意充分推开膀胱，避免膀胱损伤的可能。术野暴露较困难，要求术者熟练掌握阴式手术的操作技巧，对于憩室的正确定位很大程度上依赖于术者的经验；腹腔镜手术缝合时组织对合困难。因此需要由有丰富经阴道和腹腔镜手术经验的医师进行操作。

（6）术后阴道流血时间长，15~20天不等，术后使用抗生素预防感染；术后禁盆浴、性生活1个月。如出现阴道流血量多于月经量、发热、阴道脓性分泌物等症状时应及时就诊。术后需随访治疗效果，如果术后3个月仍无效，建议进一步寻找病因，比如是否存在子宫内膜增殖症或者子宫内膜不规则脱落，并进行相应治疗。

（7）CSD修补手术后再次妊娠的时间：对于行剖宫产术后子宫瘢痕切除术治疗的患者，由于子宫切口的最佳愈合时间为术后2～4年，故建议术后避孕2年；而对于腹腔镜下"折叠对接缝合法"及宫腔镜手术者，由于没有破坏子宫的完整性，可适当缩短避孕时间，在术后6个月可酌情计划妊娠。

（三）诊治流程（图4-1）

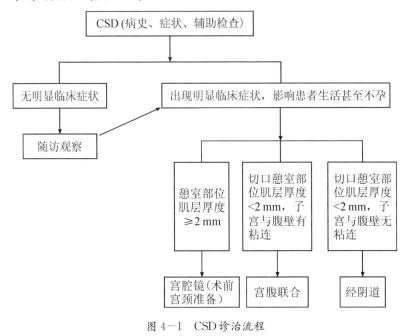

图4-1　CSD诊治流程

张建平　唐溪瞳

【参考文献】

[1] 中华医学会计划生育分会. 剖宫产术后子宫瘢痕憩室诊治专家共识[J]. 中华妇产科杂志，2019，54（3）：145-148.

[2] 李健，白文佩. 剖宫产切口愈合不良的治疗方法[J]. 国际妇产科杂志，2017，44（5）：543-546.

[3] 陈雨柔，张蔚，刘福林，等. 宫腹腔镜联合手术与经阴式手术比较治疗剖宫产切口憩室的Meta分析[J]. 现代妇产科进展，2016，25（9）：667-672.

[4] 罗蒲英，凌燕，彭诗维. 剖宫产术后子宫切口憩室的微创手术方式探讨[J]. 中国妇幼保健，2014，29（30）：5004-5006.

[5] 张宁宁，王光伟，杨清. 腹腔镜下不同方法修复剖宫产子宫瘢痕憩室的

临床疗效分析 [J]. 中国医科大学学报，2017，46（9）：853-856.

[6] 张燕茹，黄惠娟. 剖宫产术后子宫切口憩室的诊治进展 [J]. 中国计划生育学杂志，2017，25（7）：494-501.

[7] 赵琪锦，李楚，杨云萍. 子宫瘢痕憩室的研究进展 [J]. 中国计划生育学杂志，2022，30（9）：21565-21569.

[8] TOWER A M，FRISHMAN G N. Cesarean scar defects：an underrecognized cause of abnormal uterine bleeding and other gynecologic complications [J]. J Minim Invasive Gynecol，2013，20（5）：562-572.

[9] 李丽萍，刘杰，陆相辉. 宫腹腔镜下瘢痕切除修补术与雌孕激素治疗78 例剖宫产切口憩室的效果比较研究 [J]. 中国妇幼保健，2015，30（25）：4407-4409.

[10] CHANG Y，TSAI E M，LONG C Y，et al. Resectoscopic treatment combined with sonohysterographic evaluation of women with postmenstrual bleeding as a result of previous cesarean delivery scar defects [J]. Am J Obstet Gynecol，2009，200（4）：370. e1-370. e4.

[11] TANIMURA S，FUNAMOTO H，HOSONO T，et al. New diagnostic criteria and operative strategy for cesarean scar syndrome：endoscopic repair for secondary infertility caused by cesarean scar defect [J]. J Obstet Gynaecol Res，2015，41（9）：1363-1369.

[12] LI C，GUO Y，LIU Y，et al. Hysteroscopic and laparoscopic management of uterine defects on previous cesarean delivery scars [J]. J Perinat Med，2014，42（3）：363-370.

[13] 张彤艳，张学强，张宁，等. 腹腔镜子宫下段肌层折叠缝合联合宫腔镜治疗剖宫产术后子宫瘢痕憩室的临床效果观察 [J]. 中国临床新医学，2021，14（12）：1192-1195.

[14] BDOUR H AL M，IBTEHAL A. Hysteroscopy in the treatment of myometrial scar defect（diverticulum）following cesarean section delivery：a systematic review and meta-analysis [J]. Cureus，2020，12（11）：11317.

[15] ABACJEW-CHMYLKO A，DARIUSZ G W，HANNA O. Hysteroscopy in the treatment of uterine cesarean section scar diverticulum：a systematic review [J]. Adv Med Sci，2017，62（2）：230-239.

第五章　妊娠残留物的诊治流程及手术操作规范

胚物残留（retained products of conception，RPOC）是指在流产或分娩后部分胚胎或胎盘组织残留在宫腔内，多数需要手术清除，可能引起腹痛、出血及感染，继而引起宫腔粘连、闭经、继发不孕等。宫腔镜对于宫腔内病变的观察一目了然，对于宫腔内妊娠残留物，可在宫腔镜下诊断定位与治疗。

一、诊断

1. 病史：有流产或分娩史；排除再次妊娠。

2. 临床症状：可能有阴道流血持续不净、月经未复潮或伴有感染症状，也可无症状。

3. 体格检查：子宫正常大小或增大，合并感染可出现压痛。

4. 辅助检查：

（1）超声检查提示宫内不均质异常回声；HCG 检查为阳性或正常。

（2）宫腔镜检查：宫腔镜下见宫腔内有局限性的灰黄色或暗紫色不规则的机化组织与子宫壁粘连。

二、鉴别诊断

1. 子宫内膜息肉：多表现为经期延长、经间期出血、经量增多或不规则出血，超声提示宫腔内稍高回声或不均质区，宫腔镜及病检可明确诊断。

2. 异位妊娠：有停经、腹痛、阴道流血，HCG 阳性，超声提示宫腔内未见孕囊，附件区混合回声包块。

3. 滋养细胞疾病：有停经史，阴道无或有不规则流血，血 HCG 水平异常。完全性葡萄胎的超声图像表现为宫腔内充满不均质密集状或短条状回声，呈"落雪状"，水泡较大时则呈"蜂窝状"。部分性葡萄胎可在胎盘部位出现由局灶性水泡状胎块引起的超声图像改变，有时还可见胎儿及羊膜腔。滋养细胞肿瘤子宫正常大小或不同程度增大，肌层内可见高回声团，边界清或不清，无包膜，也可表现为整个子宫呈弥漫性增高回声，多普勒显示有丰富的血流信号和低阻力型血流频谱。CT 或 MRI 可发现转移病灶。

三、治疗

1. 宫腔镜手术适应证：

（1）宫腔妊娠残留物或伴有异常子宫出血。

（2）宫腔深度≤12 cm。

2. 麻醉选择：静脉麻醉或者硬膜外椎管内麻醉。

3. 手术时机：经观察或者药物治疗后，HCG 下降及超声血流明显减弱。不建议出血多时手术，极易因为血窦开放出现空气栓塞及水中毒。

（1）无宫腔感染征象：多数专家建议无感染征象，胚物残留 6～8 周时宫腔镜手术去除。

（2）合并宫腔感染征象：阴道流血量少，需抗感染治疗 24～48 小时后再行手术；阴道流血量多，需抗感染的同时进行手术治疗。感染严重时应先夹取大块组织，避免搔刮宫腔，待感染被控制后再次清宫。

4. 术前准备：

（1）术前 2 天分次口服米非司酮（有米非司酮禁忌证除外）共 150 mg 或顿服米非司酮 200 mg，术前 4～6 小时阴道后穹隆放置米索前列醇 0.4 mg 或卡孕栓 1 mg（有米索前列醇禁忌证除外）软化宫颈，促进子宫收缩。

（2）对于胚物残留时间长、机化的或已经存在宫腔粘连，或在既往有多次人工流产手术史且有生育要求者，可以在术前 3～5 天开始使用戊酸雌二醇片 2 mg，每天 2 次，以提高子宫平滑肌对缩宫素的敏感性，松弛宫口，增强子宫收缩力和促进内膜的生长，术后可以继续促内膜生长治疗。

5. 手术操作步骤：

（1）经宫腔镜残留妊娠物清宫术手术操作规范：

1）患者取膀胱截石位，外阴、阴道常规消毒铺单。

2）Hegar 扩宫器扩张宫颈口至 7 号，连接宫腔镜诊断系统，缓慢置入宫腔镜，按顺序观察子宫底及子宫前、后、左、右壁，再检查子宫角及输卵管开口，观察子宫腔的形态、子宫内膜有无异常及妊娠残留物的部位和量，最后缓慢退出镜体，退镜过程中检视宫颈内口和宫颈管。

3）经宫腔镜明确诊断，确定残留部位后，取出宫腔镜，如果残留物少、组织疏松，直接用宫腔镜电切环（不带电）将残留物带出，对与子宫壁粘连致密的少许胎盘组织则用微型钳夹出；如果大量胎盘组织残留，可先予以取物钳或者卵圆钳钳取，与子宫壁粘连致密的部分则改用外径 10 mm 的电切镜切除胎盘组织。如果未清除干净，可重复操作，直至残留物清除干净为止。

（2）宫腔组织机械性旋切术手术操作流程：

1）常规外阴、阴道消毒，宫颈扩张至 Hager 7 号。

2）将宫腔组织机械性旋切装置的真空负压根据膨宫液的进出平衡原则设定在 250～350 mmHg（33.3～46.7 kPa）之间，膨宫机压力需设定在 80～100 mmHg（10.7～13.3 kPa），流速调至 500 mL/min。

3）经宫腔镜工作通道置入组织切除装置进行手术操作。将机械旋宫腔组织旋切装置的切割窗直接紧贴胚胎残留物表面，在残留物表面来回"扫"，当组织残留物少并紧贴宫壁时，切除装置的切割窗最好距离残留物附着处 3～5 mm，或者用微型钳钳夹宫壁的残留物，避免切割窗切割时损伤残留物下方的内膜及肌层。重复操作，直至残留物清除干净为止。

6. 术中术后注意事项：

（1）对于宫腔≥12 cm 的妊娠残留物的患者，如果没有合并感染，可待子宫复旧好，子宫腔缩小后再行宫腔镜直视下清宫术，以减少遍刮宫腔导致内膜损伤。

（2）术中注意用宫缩剂加强宫缩，在宫缩好的情况下宫腔形态轮廓更清楚，能减少术中出血。术前可用缩宫素 10 U 宫颈注射，如果术中宫缩欠佳可加用麦角新碱 0.2 mg 宫颈注射，或者稀释后垂体后叶素 3～6 U 宫颈注射，或者肛门内上卡孕栓 1 mg 或者米索前列醇 0.4 mg。

（3）注意保护避免损伤胚物着床部位下方和无胚物着床部位的子宫内膜。尽量在宫腔镜直视下取出妊娠残留物，避免伤及子宫基底层及损失邻近子宫内膜。与宫壁粘连致密时用环状电极在其不带电的情况下钝性逆行推，分离组织与子宫的粘连，切除妊娠残留物时需要降低电切频率（220～240 W）；用机械旋切时，可用切割器的头端钝性分离组织与宫壁的粘连，尽量让残留组织游离，接近宫壁时切割窗不要紧贴残留物附着面。

（4）宫腔镜手术中发现有宫腔粘连，对于中央性粘连，予以分离后手术，以利于妊娠残留物完整彻底清除，对于周围型粘连，待患者恢复月经后再行宫腔粘连分离术，清宫术中可宫腔内放置交联透明质酸钠防粘连，术后需要用雌激素促内膜生长等治疗。

（5）如清宫术后出血多，加强宫缩同时可采用水囊压迫，将 Foley 尿管头端剪除后置入宫腔，在超声引导下，往囊内注入生理盐水，超声下见水囊完全紧贴宫腔面，引流管内无活动性血液流出后即可。

7. 诊治流程（图 5-1）：

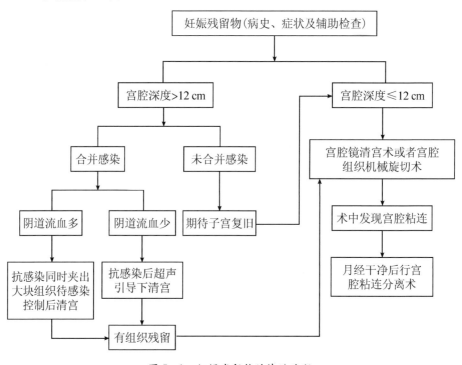

图 5-1　妊娠残留物的诊治流程

罗婕

【参考文献】

[1] 付凤仙，段华. B超联合宫腔镜在宫内妊娠组织残留诊断和治疗中的临床价值 [J]. 中国微创外科杂志，2011，11（9）：797－800.

[2] 徐大宝，薛敏. 宫腔镜在不全流产诊治中的价值 [J]. 中国内镜杂志，2004，10（3）：38－40.

[3] 卢艳，崔超美，李雪英. 美奥舒宫内组织切除系统在产后胎盘残留的临床应用价值 [J]. 湖南师范大学学报（医学版），2017，14（3）：46－47.

[4] 贾柠伊，冯力民. 宫腔镜应用于胚物残留治疗的意义 [J]. 中国计划生育和妇产科，2015，7（10）：8－10.

[5] Jose Hidalgo lopez. HTRs：first steps to the end of blind intrauterine procedures-key aspects of an epic congresss [J]. Hysteroscopy Newsletter vol 8 Issue 3 P. 3－6.

[6] 谢幸，孔北华，段涛. 妇产科学 [M]. 9版. 北京：人民卫生出版社，2018.

第六章　子宫畸形的
诊治流程及手术操作规范

子宫畸形为常见的女性生殖系统发育异常，是胚胎在 6～18 周时双侧副中肾管发育、融合或吸收异常所致，不同阶段、不同程度的发育或融合、吸收障碍会导致不同类型的子宫畸形，但其确切的发病机制仍待进一步研究。不同文献报道的子宫畸形在人群中的患病率差异较大（0.16%～10%），在高风险人群如不孕、复发性流产女性中患病率通常较高。

一、诊断

1. 临床症状：根据子宫畸形的程度而有不同的临床表现。有些子宫畸形患者可无任何症状，月经、生育均无异常表现，仅在体检或妇科手术时偶被发现，但亦有些患者表现为月经异常、痛经、性生活困难、不孕、习惯性流产。先天性无子宫、始基子宫患者无月经，幼稚子宫患者可无月经或月经过少，子宫畸形可致痛经、不孕、习惯性流产、胎位异常等。故凡有原发闭经、性生活困难、不孕、反复流产、死胎、早产、胎位异常的患者，应想到有子宫畸形之可能。

2. 体格检查：

（1）全身一般检查：注意第二性征的发育情况，如身材、体态及乳房的发育是否正常，以排除有无性腺发育异常。

（2）妇科检查：妇科检查时注意有无双阴道、双宫颈，子宫大小、形态、位置有无异常。

3. 辅助检查：

（1）影像学检查：影像学检查的主要目的为提示生殖器官畸形的部位，局部解剖特点，是否存在相关合并症，以及排查有无合并其他器官形态学异常。盆腔超声检查因无创、费用低廉，应为第一步的检查方法。MRI 检查具有无创、软组织分辨率高、多参数、多平面和多方位成像的特点，还可以进行三维图像重建，能清楚显示宫底外形轮廓和宫腔结构，同时能观察并发的其他病变，如泌尿系统畸形、附件区疾病等，是诊断子宫畸形且区分畸形类型的理想的检查方法。另外，在 MRI 图像中临床医生可以对子宫畸形的各项指标进行定量分析，如双侧宫角内膜连线、双侧内膜夹角、宫底部凹陷深度、纵隔长度等，诊断准确度高达 100％。但相较于超声，MRI 价格较昂贵，设备复杂，一定程度上限制了其临床应用。

（2）子宫输卵管造影（HSG）：可以显示宫腔和输卵管的位置、形态、大小，能够较好地显示大部分的宫腔发育异常，是协助诊断子宫畸形的主要方法，有其他辅助检查不可替代的优势。但 HSG 不能显示子宫肌层及外部轮廓，为有创操作，患者暴露于射线，并且对于诊断细微的子宫畸形敏感度较低，目前很少单独用于诊断子宫畸形。

（3）实验室检查：特殊的实验室检查包括染色体检查及女性激素水平检查，必要时需通过有关下丘脑、垂体、肾上腺皮质功能的检查来协助诊断。

（4）内镜检查：对于合并有其他手术治疗指征，经上述辅助检查仍不能完全明确诊断者，可考虑通过腹腔镜或宫腔镜检查进行诊断并同时完成治疗。对于少数合并下泌尿道（尿道、膀胱）畸形的患者，膀胱镜检查有利于协助其诊断。

二、分类

1988 年，美国生育协会（American Fertility Society，AFS）修订的女性生殖器官畸形分类系统，目前在世界范围内被广泛接受，普遍应用于临床。根据米勒管发育异常的发生阶段，又进一步将子宫发育异常分成 7 种不同的类型。Ⅰ型，不同程度的子宫发育不全或缺失；Ⅱ型，单角子宫、残角子宫（一侧中肾旁管发育不全或者缺失）；Ⅲ型，双子宫（中肾旁管未融合，各自发育成子宫和阴道；Ⅳ型，双角子宫（宫角在宫底水平融合不全）；Ⅴ型，纵隔子宫（子宫阴道纵隔未吸收或吸收不全）；Ⅵ型，弓形子宫（宫底有一轻微凹陷，源于近乎完全吸收的子宫阴道纵隔）；Ⅶ型，己烯雌酚（diethylstilbestrol，DES）相关异常（胎儿期在宫内受 DES 暴露可引起子宫肌层形成收缩带样发育异常，宫腔呈 T 形改变）。见表6-1。

表 6-1　美国生育协会（AFS）的子宫畸形分类

类型	描述	解剖图示
Ⅰ	不同程度的子宫发育不全或缺失	a. 阴道发育不全　b. 宫颈发育不全 c. 仅有宫底　d. 双侧输卵管未发育　e. 复合型
Ⅱ	单角子宫、残角子宫	a. 宫腔互通　b. 宫腔不通 c. 无宫腔残角子宫　d. 单角子宫
Ⅲ	双子宫	
Ⅳ	双角子宫	a. 完全性　b. 部分性
Ⅴ	纵隔子宫	a. 完全性　b. 部分性
Ⅵ	弓形子宫	
Ⅶ	己烯雌酚相关异常	

1998 年，AFS 进一步完善了子宫颈、阴道、外生殖器畸形的分类（表 6-2）。

表 6-2　子宫颈、阴道、外生殖器畸形的分类

畸形总称	分类	亚类
子宫颈畸形	子宫颈未发育	
	子宫颈完全闭锁	
	子宫颈管狭窄	
	子宫颈角度异常	
	先天性子宫颈延长症伴子宫颈管狭窄	
	双子宫颈等子宫颈发育异常	
阴道畸形	副中肾管发育不良（MRKH 综合征）	阴道闭锁 Ⅱ 型
	泌尿生殖窦发育不良	阴道闭锁 Ⅰ 型
	副中肾管垂直融合异常	完全性阴道横隔
		不完全性阴道横隔
	副中肾管侧面融合异常	完全性阴道纵隔
		部分性阴道纵隔
	副中肾管垂直-侧面融合异常	阴道斜隔
外生殖器畸形	处女膜闭锁（无孔处女膜）	
	外生殖器男性化	

2013 年 6 月，欧洲人类生殖与胚胎学会（ESHRE）和欧洲妇科内镜学会（ESGE）发布了新的女性生殖器官畸形分类共识，以解剖学为基础，将最常见也最重要的子宫畸形分为 7 个主型，各主型根据临床意义又分为不同亚型（表 6-3），子宫颈及阴道的畸形单独根据临床意义分为不同亚型（表 6-4）。

表 6－3　欧洲人类生殖与胚胎学会及欧洲妇科内镜学会子宫畸形分类

类型	描述	亚类	解剖图示
U0	正常子宫		
U1	子宫形态异常	a. T 形子宫	
		b. 幼稚子宫	
		c. 其他子宫发育不良	
U2	纵隔子宫	a. 部分纵隔子宫（宫底内陷＜宫壁厚度的 50％且宫腔内隔厚度＞宫壁厚度的 50％）	
		b. 完全纵隔子宫（宫底内陷＜宫壁厚度的 50％）	
U3	双角子宫	a. 部分双角子宫（宫底内陷＞宫壁厚度的 50％）	
		b. 完全双角子宫	
		c. 双角纵隔子宫（宫底内陷＞宫壁厚度的 50％且宫腔内隔厚度＞宫壁厚度的 150％）	
U4	单角子宫	a. 对侧伴有宫腔的残角子宫（与单角子宫相通或不相通）	

续表

类型	描述	亚类	解剖图示
		b. 对侧为无宫腔残角子宫或缺如	
U5	发育不良	a. 有宫腔始基子宫（双侧或单侧）	
		b. 无宫腔始基子宫（双侧或一侧子宫残基，或无子宫）	
U6	未分类畸形		

表 6-4　欧洲人类生殖与胚胎学会及欧洲妇科内镜学会子宫颈及阴道畸形分类

类型	描述
C0	正常子宫颈
C1	纵隔子宫颈
C2	双（正常）子宫颈
C3	一侧子宫颈发育不良
C4	（单个）子宫颈发育不良
	子宫颈未发育
	子宫颈完全闭锁
	子宫颈外口闭塞
	条索状子宫颈
	子宫颈残迹
V0	正常阴道
V1	非梗阻性阴道纵隔
V2	梗阻性阴道纵隔
V3	阴道横隔和（或）处女膜闭锁
V4	阴道闭锁

三、治疗

子宫畸形的治疗原则是解除梗阻，恢复正常的解剖结构和生理功能，提供生育条件和提高生命质量。

1. 手术指征：子宫畸形明确诊断后，应根据患者的临床症状、生育要求及既往孕产史等因素决定个体化的治疗方案。

先天性无子宫、始基子宫、幼稚子宫患者终身无受孕可能，无须手术。有生育要求者，若无不良孕产史，可先试孕，妊娠失败率达 70% 左右。但如何预测这类患者今后是否会有流产、胎位异常、早产等不良孕产情况，是否在不良孕产发生之前行手术治疗存在争议。宫腔镜成形术的手术适应证为超声、宫腔镜检查或宫腹腔镜联合检查可疑或诊断为子宫畸形，并有以下一项症状者：

（1）有自然流产史 2 次以上，或者原因不明的不孕症。

（2）需辅助生育技术的原发性不孕症。

（3）有宫腔积血、周期性腹痛或急腹症症状。

因妊娠期手术更易发生宫腔粘连、出血、感染等并发症，不建议在流产等妊娠物清除术同时行子宫畸形矫治术。

2. 麻醉选择：硬膜外麻醉或静脉麻醉，或全身麻醉。

3. 手术时机：月经干净 3～7 天，有梗阻性症状时做。

4. 术前准备：

（1）病情告知与知情选择：对于无不良孕产患者，可试孕；但关于如何预测这类患者今后是否会有流产、胎位异常、早产等不良孕产情况，是否在不良孕产发生之前行手术治疗仍存在争议。告知如果妊娠，有 70% 的妊娠可能结局不良。

（2）宫颈准备：术前晚放置扩张棒扩张或宫颈备管或阴道上药［米索前列醇 0.4 mg 或卡孕栓 1 mg（排除米索前列醇禁忌证）］软化宫颈。对于双宫颈完全纵隔子宫者，一般建议术前 2～3 天即开始用米索前列醇片或卡孕栓 0.4 mg，每天 1 次，放置阴道内。

（3）术前禁食 6 小时以上。

四、几种子宫畸形手术操作规范

（一）T 型子宫手术操作规范

1. 患者取膀胱截石位，丙泊酚静脉麻醉，外阴、阴道常规消毒铺单。

Hegar 扩宫器扩张宫颈口至 7 号。

2. 连接宫腔镜诊断系统，缓慢置入宫腔镜，按顺序观察子宫底及子宫前、后、左、右壁，再检查子宫角及输卵管开口，观察宫腔狭窄，两角较深，与宫体呈"T"形。

3. 再次扩张宫颈至 10 号，用针状电极小心地从双侧宫角至峡部垂直划开或切除子宫侧壁过多的肌层，切割深度不超过 5~7 mm（一个针状电极的深度为 3 mm），越向下方深度逐渐减少，薄化子宫壁，扩大宫腔的容积，修整宫腔形态至基本正常。

（二）纵隔子宫

目前，超声监护或腹腔镜监护宫腔镜子宫纵隔切开术仍然是治疗纵隔子宫的标准术式，可采用电切法和剪刀法，切开纵隔、恢复宫腔形态和生殖功能是手术成功的标准。针状电极切开子宫纵隔是最常用的手术方法。

1. 子宫不全纵隔电切术手术操作规范：

（1）患者取膀胱截石位，丙泊酚静脉麻醉，外阴、阴道常规消毒铺单。Hegar 扩宫器扩张宫颈口至 7 号。

（2）连接宫腔镜诊断系统，缓慢置入宫腔镜，按顺序观察子宫底及子宫前、后、左、右壁，以及纵隔的起始部位。在宫颈内口上方，再检查双侧子宫角及输卵管开口，观察宫腔内膜情况，有无合并宫腔粘连及息肉等，以及输卵管开口是否可见。

（3）再次扩张宫颈至 10 号，沿着双侧输卵管开口的连线方向水平切开，用电切镜针状电极自隔板末端小心前推，分离隔板，再交替自一侧向对侧横向划开隔板，直至宫底部，如果隔板比较狭长，也可采用环形电极自纵隔末端一侧开始，向另一侧切割隔板，然后自另一侧向回切割，重复切割操作，达宫底部。隔板切净时可见宫底纵形排列的肌纤维，其间裂隙状的血窦及邻近的子宫角和输卵管开口。

（4）手术结束时两侧宫腔打通，形成一个对称的倒三角形宫腔。

2. 子宫不全纵隔冷刀切除术手术操作规范：

（1）患者取膀胱截石位，丙泊酚静脉麻醉，外阴、阴道常规消毒铺单。Hegar 扩宫器扩张宫颈口至 7 号。

（2）连接宫腔镜诊断系统，缓慢置入宫腔镜，按顺序观察子宫底及子宫前、后、左、右壁，以及纵隔的起始部位。在宫颈内口上方，再检查双侧子宫角及输卵管开口，观察宫腔内膜情况，有无合并宫腔粘连及息肉等，以及输卵管开口是否可见。

（3）从纵隔末端开始，沿着双侧输卵管开口的连线方向水平，以剪刀横向左右交替剪开纵隔，重复操作，直至达宫底纵隔基底部，有明显出血的患者可用汽化电极电凝止血。

徐大宝教授发明了标记法，先在宫底的左右侧与双侧输卵管在同一水平线上的位置，需要切除纵隔终止的位置剪开一刀作为最终结束手术前的标记，剪开隔板时宫底部到了标记部位即停止手术。也可采用宫腔机械旋切器，切割窗紧贴纵隔，从隔板末端开始，在纵隔表面反复地"啃食"纵隔组织，直至隔板完全被啃食，达宫底纵隔基底部。隔板切净时可见宫底纵形排列的肌纤维、其间裂隙状的血窦及邻近的子宫角和输卵管开口。

（4）手术结束时两侧宫腔打通，形成一个对称的倒三角形宫腔。降低膨宫压力，手术切开部位无明显出血即可结束手术。

3. 子宫完全纵隔电切术手术操作规范：

（1）患者取膀胱截石位，丙泊酚静脉麻醉，外阴、阴道常规消毒铺单。Hegar扩宫器扩张宫颈口至7号。

（2）连接宫腔镜诊断系统，缓慢置入宫腔镜，按顺序观察子宫底及子宫前、后、左、右壁，以及纵隔的起始部位；观察双侧宫角及输卵管开口；观察宫腔内膜情况，有无合并宫腔粘连及息肉等，以及输卵管开口是否可见。

（3）观察宫腔内的完全纵隔的特征，选择切开纵隔的起始部位：

1）部分患者起始部位在内口下方，但在宫颈内口上方可见部分纵隔吸收，形成小的缺失使两侧宫腔相通；可以利用此处纵隔缺失处为起点，针状电极向头侧方向切开纵隔隔板直到宫底部。

2）对于完全纵隔子宫没有纵隔缺失形成两侧宫腔不相通，可采用球囊法作为指示；首先选择宫腔较大、宫颈较优侧置入宫腔镜，然后将输卵管通液管置入对侧宫腔，将3~5 mL生理盐水反复推注、抽吸，使得完全纵隔的下段向置入宫腔镜的一侧的宫腔膨出和回缩，协助判断宫腔镜贯穿切开完全纵隔的位置和方向；用针状电极在子宫下段、宫颈内口上方的纵隔内凸部位切开纵隔，直至可见对侧宫腔的球囊，两侧宫腔贯通后取出球囊；然后按照部分纵隔子宫的手术方法切开纵隔。

（4）手术结束时两侧宫腔打通，形成一个对称的倒三角形宫腔。

4. Robert 子宫宫腔镜手术操作规范：

（1）患者取膀胱截石位，丙泊酚静脉麻醉，外阴、阴道常规消毒铺单。Hegar 扩宫器扩张宫颈口至 7 号。

（2）连接宫腔镜诊断系统，缓慢置入宫腔镜，按顺序观察子宫底及子宫前、后、左、右壁，以及隔板的起始部位；观察双侧宫角及输卵管开口是否可见；观察宫腔内膜情况，有无合并宫腔粘连及息肉等，以及输卵管开口是否可见。

（3）超声监护下宫腔镜下于隔板薄弱处，自一侧宫腔用针状电极横行打开隔板，并向上下分别切开完全隔板，封闭侧宫腔流出褐色黏稠血液和黄褐色渣样组织，完全流净后见隔板侧的输卵管开口，必要时可电切多余的隔板。

（4）手术结束时观察子宫腔为一个对称的倒三角形。

（三）双角子宫

1. 不完全双角纵隔子宫宫腹腔镜联合手术操作规范：

（1）患者取膀胱截石位，丙泊酚静脉麻醉，外阴、阴道常规消毒铺单。Hegar 扩宫器扩张宫颈口至 7 号。

（2）连接宫腔镜诊断系统，缓慢置入宫腔镜，按顺序观察子宫底及子宫前、后、左、右壁，以及纵隔的起始部位；观察双侧宫角及输卵管开口；观察宫腔、宫颈管内膜情况，有无合并宫腔粘连及息肉等，以及双侧输卵管开口是否可见；隔板的起始部位的位置，超声监测隔板、宫底肌层以及其他部位肌层的厚度。

（3）超声监护下宫腔镜下环形电极切割，或针状电极划开宫腔的隔板组织及宫底增厚的肌壁组织，至宫底厚度与其他宫壁均匀一致。

（4）术后宫腔镜观察宫腔形态呈双侧宫角稍深、宫底稍向内凹陷的倒三角形。

2. 完全双角子宫宫腹腔镜联合手术操作规范：

（1）采用全身麻醉，先行腹腔镜探查术，观察盆腔情况及宫底外形，明确诊断。然后在腹腔镜监护下，宫颈扩张棒逐次扩张宫颈至 10.5 号，膨宫压力 100 mmHg（13.3kPa）。

（2）置入宫腔镜，按顺序观察子宫颈与子宫体、隔板及双侧输卵管开口状态、子宫各壁及子宫腔、宫颈管内膜等。

（3）用等离子针状双极电切划开子宫隔板，打开子宫底正中肌壁，切至子宫底正中浆膜层，形成人工穿孔，子宫底完全与腹腔相通。

（4）然后在腹腔镜下用单极电针横向打开宫底，子宫底横行切开至距双侧子宫角内 1.5 cm 处。

（5）用 0 号可吸收线 8 字缝合黏膜下浅肌层，闭合宫腔。肌层间断 8 字缝合，浆肌层纵向间断内翻缝合共 5~11 针，形成一个正常形态的子宫。

（四）单角子宫宫腔镜下子宫壁切开术（transcervical uterine incision，TCUI）

1. 患者取膀胱截石位，丙泊酚静脉麻醉，外阴、阴道常规消毒铺单。Hegar 扩宫器扩张宫颈口至 7 号。

2. 连接宫腔镜诊断系统，缓慢置入宫腔镜，按顺序观察子宫底及子宫前、后、左、右壁；观察宫腔、宫颈管内膜情况，有无合并宫腔粘连及息肉等，以及单个输卵管开口位置。单角子宫宫腔镜下表现为宫腔呈单角状，或呈长梭形，仅见一侧宫角及输卵管开口。

3. 在超声监护下宫腔镜下环形电极切割或针状电极，首先横向切除或切开肌壁，宫腔电切镜切除或切开肌壁的深度，在宫底和上段宫腔部位达 1 cm 以上，形成新的 2 cm 以上宽度的宫底，然后纵向自上而下，上深下浅，切除或切开单侧宫角对侧的肌壁，长约 4 cm，可扩大子宫容积。

4. 术毕形成倒三角形上段较为宽阔的宫腔。

5. 无功能的残角子宫如果在宫角部与单角子宫紧贴，可充分利用非单角侧无功能的残角肥厚的肌壁组织，扩大宫腔容积，无功能的残角子宫可行输卵管切除术；有功能的残角子宫如果与单角子宫相距较远，需行腹腔镜残角子宫及输卵管切除术，或仅切除残角侧的部分子宫肌壁及子宫内膜和输卵管，以保留残角侧的子宫动脉和子宫卵巢供血；有功能的残角子宫如果与单角子宫紧贴，也有将有功能残角与单角子宫在宫腹腔镜联合下融合成新的宫腔的报道。

（五）宫腔镜弓形子宫及鞍状子宫成形术

1. 患者取膀胱截石位，丙泊酚静脉麻醉，外阴、阴道常规消毒铺单。Hegar 扩宫器扩张宫颈口至 7 号。

2. 连接宫腔镜诊断系统，缓慢置入宫腔镜，按顺序观察子宫底及子宫前、后、左、右壁，双侧宫角及输卵管开口；可见宫底宽厚、内凸，但无明确隔板。

超声监测宫底肌层的厚度。

3. 超声监护下宫腔镜下针状电极适度划开宫底部浅层肌壁，每次较浅切割，并修整两侧近宫角部创面，使其形成平坦的子宫底。

4. 腹腔镜下弓形子宫宫底浆膜面大致正常，有时略宽平，但无明显凹陷。鞍状子宫的宫底有明显凹陷。

（六）子宫畸形术中术后注意事项

1. 子宫纵隔切除术中及术后注意事项：

（1）准确判断手术终止时机。切开纵隔至近宫底部时，需要准确判断手术终止的时机。术前三维或者四维超声显示宫底的外形，必要时术中使用腹腔镜监测，可以准确观察子宫底外形。完全切除子宫纵隔的标准是宫底部肌层的厚度恢复为正常子宫肌壁的厚度，而不是宫腔形态是否恢复为倒三角形；纵隔组织致密且基本不含血管，而宫底的肌层呈网格状、粉红色且含有血管，该特点在宫腔镜术中也可协助判断纵隔是否已经完全切除或者是否已经切除过深且达到宫底肌层。

当宫底外形正常时，宫腔镜下切除纵隔至宫腔内宫底形态与正常宫腔形态相同即可。也就是说，宫底的内轮廓呈稍弧形凸向宫腔，其最凸向宫腔的部分大约低于双侧输卵管口连线水平 0.5 cm。

当宫底外形不像正常宫底呈弧形稍凸向宫腔外，而是呈平的，这时宫腔镜纵隔切除应当于宫底呈弧形凸向宫腔最明显处在双侧输卵管口连线水平约 1 cm 时停止手术。

当宫底外形凹陷向宫腔方向，宫腔镜下纵隔切除应当于宫底内轮廓呈弧形凸向宫腔最明显处在双侧输卵管口连线水平下 ［1 cm＋宫底外形凹陷向宫腔的深度（cm）］左右时停止手术。

（2）双宫颈完全性纵隔子宫宫颈部分的纵隔不能切除，避免宫颈功能不全。合并阴道纵隔不影响性生活及分娩者无须切除阴道纵隔。

（3）子宫纵隔切开术后 1～3 个月经周期且月经干净后 3～7 天复查宫腔镜，明确是否有宫腔粘连、残留纵隔等，术后有时可见子宫底部有残留隔板，只要其长度＜0.5 cm，可不处理。若残留隔板较长，或宫腔内形成粘连，可行二次宫腔镜手术切除。

2. 双角子宫术中术后注意事项：

（1）双角子宫的宫腹腔镜诊断：腹腔镜下双角子宫的宫底浆膜面横径宽，两侧宫角远离，宫底正中有不同程度凹陷。宫腔镜着重观察两侧宫腔分离位置。宫腔镜下可见两侧略狭长宫腔，宫腔顶端可见单侧输卵管开口，两侧宫腔分离位置可在宫腔上段、中段或下段，未达宫颈内口水平。两侧宫腔分离在宫腔上段者为不完全双角子宫，宫底肌层厚度一致。不完全双角纵隔子宫，宫底内陷大于宫壁厚度的 50％，且宫腔内隔板厚度大于宫壁厚度的 150％，隔板在中段和下段者为完全性双角子宫。

（2）宫腹腔镜完全双角子宫融合术需要术者有熟练的宫腹腔镜手术技巧，术中要精密缝合子宫肌层前后壁，以免妊娠时子宫破裂。

3. 单角子宫宫腹腔镜联合子宫壁切开术：夏恩兰等分析 2010 年 1 月至 2014 年 12 月该院诊治单角子宫不孕患者 33 例，随访 10~70 个月，术后妊娠 20 例，15 例成功分娩并获活婴。与术前比较，自然流产率、足月分娩率、获活婴率均较术前有明显改善；可作为单角子宫合并不孕症患者成形的推荐术式。畸形子宫的宫颈肌肉成分增加，结缔组织减少，宫颈不足以对抗妊娠后增加的不对称的宫腔压力，而致流产、早产。据报道，先天性子宫畸形的宫颈功能不全发生率为 30％，多篇文献报道有中期妊娠流产史的单角子宫患者通过宫颈环扎提高了胎儿存活率。因此，对单角子宫的治疗，还应关注宫颈功能不全的问题。

4. 子宫畸形矫治术中术后出血：电切术中小血管出血及手术结束前降低膨宫压力检查有出血部位，均可用电凝止血；术后如果出血较多，可能存在子宫收缩不良，或者术中血管回缩所致，可宫颈注射宫缩剂，并宫腔内置入 Foley 尿管囊内注入生理盐水 3~5 mL，一般均能止血。

5. 术中要预防子宫穿孔：术中一般采用超声监护或者超声和腹腔镜监护，超声下见浆膜下血肿，灌流液进入腹腔，宫腔镜下见到腹腔组织或器官等均提示子宫穿孔，如腹腔镜下见浆膜层起气泡或者透光试验不均匀都提示子宫宫底切割过度，是子宫穿孔的先兆，需要立即停止手术。

6. 子宫畸形合并宫腔粘连：则需要子宫畸形矫治的同时，按照宫腔粘连手术的操作规范行宫腔粘连分离术，恢复患者宫腔的正常形态。

7. 子宫畸形矫治术后宫腔镜复查：这是大家公认的观点，术后宫腔镜复查准确了解宫腔形态，宫腔内膜情况，有无残留隔及宫腔粘连，术后复查时间一般为术后 1~3 个月。

8. 子宫畸形成形术后是否使用天然雌激素有争议。有学者认为应该是个体化的，对于纵隔子宫不伴有内膜损伤的患者，特别是伴有多发宫内膜局灶增生的患者，术后不需要给予雌激素治疗；而对于伴有宫内膜损伤的患者（如宫腔镜下见宫内膜腺体密度较正常稀少或者既往有多次宫腔操作病史及月经量减少者），建议术后给予雌激素治疗促进宫内膜的生长。

9. 对于术后是否放置宫内节育器（intrauterine device，IUD）或球囊，学术界颇有争议。但是多数研究认为，是否放置节育器没有显著区别。不过，如果纵隔子宫同时合并了宫腔粘连或者同时对左右侧壁凸向宫腔的部分进行了矫形手术，则需要按照宫腔粘连的原则处理。

10. 术后避孕时间：宫腹腔镜完全双角子宫融合术者术后避孕半年可试妊娠。其他宫腔镜下子宫畸形成形术后 8 周即可试妊娠。理论上说，子宫畸形矫治手术后妊娠有子宫破裂的风险，术后妊娠期间需要严密监护。

（七）诊治流程（图 6-1）

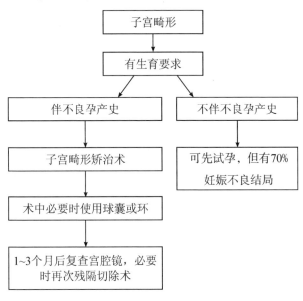

图 6-1　子宫畸形的诊治流程

李雪英　胡萃

【参考文献】

[1] 马菁苒，朱兰. 先天性子宫畸形的分类、诊断及类型鉴别［J］. 协和医

学杂志，2014，5（4）：455－459.

[2] 杨益民，黄欢，冯力民，等. 纵隔子宫诊断与治疗相关临床问题解析 [J]. 国际妇产科学杂志，2017，44（3）：248－251.

[3] 王贺，杨清，毕芳芳. 宫腔镜治疗纵隔子宫的产科结局分析 [J]. 国际妇产科学杂志，2016，43（2）：207－210.

[4] 中华医学会妇产科学分会. 女性生殖器官畸形诊治的中国专家共识 [J]. 中华妇产科杂志，2015，50（12）：881－887.

[5] 中华医学会妇产科分会. 关于女性生殖器官畸形统一命名和定义的中国专家共识 [J]. 中华妇产科杂志，2015，50（9）：648－651.

[6] 李金玉，冯力民. 宫腔镜在子宫畸形诊治中的应用现状 [J]. 中国计划生育与妇科杂志，2015，7（9）：6－11.

[7] CHAN Y Y, JAYAPRAKASAN K, ZAMORA J, et al. The prevalence of congenital uterine anomalies in unselected and high-riskpopulations：a systematic review [J]. Hum Reprod Update，2011，17（6）：761－771.

[8] 张卓颖，黄群英，孙明华，等. 磁共振成像在子宫畸形诊断中的价值 [J]. 生殖与避孕，2016，36（1）：69－73.

[9] 夏恩兰. 子宫畸形的诊治 [J]. 中国实用妇科与产科杂志，2018，34（4）：367－371.

[10] 王素敏，顾小燕，许锋. 宫腔镜子宫纵隔切开术治疗纵隔子宫 [J]. 中国实用妇科与产科杂志，2018，34（4）：371－373.

[11] 曹斌融. 常见子宫畸形的种类及诊治 [J]. 中国实用妇科与产科杂志，2005，21（8）：451－452.

[12] TOMAŽEVIČT，BAN-FRANGEŽ H，VIRANT-KLUN I，et al. Septate，subseptate and arcuate uterus decrease pregnancy and live birth rates in IVF/ICSI [J]. Reprod Biomed Online，2010，21（5）：700－705.

[13] XIA E L, LI T C, SZE-NGAR S C, et al. Reproductive outcome of transcervical uterine incision in unicornuate uterus [J]. Chin Med J（Engl），2017，130（3）：256－261.

[14] GOLAN A, LANGER R, NEUMAN M, et al. Obstetric outcome in women with congenital uterine malformations [J]. J Reprod Med，1992，37（3）：233－236.

第七章 子宫腔粘连的诊治流程及手术操作规范

子宫腔粘连（intrauterine adhesion，IUA）是妇科常见、对生育功能严重危害，并且治疗效果较差的宫腔疾病，严重影响女性生殖生理及身心健康。继1894年首次发表 IUA 的文献报道之后，1948年，Asherman 详细描述了29例流产或产后刮宫所致的 IUA 病例，并将其定义为损伤性闭经（traumatical amenorrhea），又称为阿谢曼（Asherman）综合征。目前，IUA 在我国的发病率居高不下，并且随着宫腔手术的增加呈逐年增长趋势。文献报道，妊娠相关的 IUA 占90％，非妊娠相关的约占10％，已经成为月经量减少、继发性不孕的主要原因。

一、诊断

1. 临床表现：单纯的宫颈管粘连，可引起闭经、不孕、周期性腹痛等较严重的症状；而宫腔部分或完全闭塞者，临床表现与粘连的严重程度一致，可出现月经量减少、闭经、不孕、反复流产等症状。

2. 体格检查：一般无明显异常，宫颈粘连导致宫腔积血时可出现子宫增大伴压痛。

3. 辅助检查：

（1）超声检查：二维经阴道超声（two-dimensional transvaginal ultrasound，2D-TVS）检查经济、便捷，常作为妇科病变的首选辅助检查手段，可于横断面及矢状面观察子宫腔形态、子宫内膜情况，并测量内膜厚度。IUA 最常见2D-TVS声像图表现为子宫内膜厚薄不均、边缘局部毛糙、边缘缺损、不规则、内膜线回声连续性中断，可伴不同程度宫腔积液或高回声钙化等。对于粘连范围较小，粘连带较薄，未明显影响宫腔形态及内膜完整性的轻度 IUA 易漏诊；且

2D-TVS 不能显示子宫冠状切面，故子宫底部、双侧宫角及子宫后壁粘连的检出率较低。2D-TVS 虽对诊断 IUA 具有一定价值，但单一 2D-TVS 诊断 IUA 的准确率有限。三维经阴道超声（three-dimensional transvaginal ultrasound，3D-TVS）经重建图像后可获得子宫腔冠状面的准确回声信息，整体、直观地显示包括宫颈内口及双侧宫角在内的子宫腔形态和内膜连续性，并可用于术前测量子宫内膜表面积和宫腔容积，计算粘连面积及其占宫腔总面积比例，提供粘连位置、程度及功能性子宫内膜范围等信息。IUA 冠状面 3D-TVS 声像图典型表现为宫腔两侧边内聚成角，宫腔失去正常倒三角形，内膜不同程度缺损，局部或呈低回声，宫底及两侧壁宫腔边缘不光滑。3D-TVS 可显示冠状面，这一优势能在一定程度上弥补二维超声的不足，为诊断 IUA 及其程度分级提供依据。

（2）子宫输卵管造影（HSG）：可确定宫腔粘连和封闭范围的程度。如果宫腔未完全被粘连封闭，则可显示剩余宫腔形态；如果 HSG 显示多单发或多发的充盈缺损，则诊断 IUA 较可靠。但不能提示粘连的坚韧度和类型；另外子宫充盈缺损也可由血块、气泡、子宫内膜碎片等所致，从而引起误诊。因此，临床上较少使用 HSG 作为 IUA 的诊断方法。

（3）宫腔镜：是诊断 IUA 的金标准。宫腔镜直视下检查，可确定粘连的范围、性质、部位和程度，还可应用于手术治疗后的复查。参照冯缵冲主编的《新编不孕不育治疗学》分类标准，粘连类型分为：①中央型粘连，又称桥样粘连，宫腔内可见明显的粘连带，似桥样连接宫腔左右壁或前后壁，宫腔有时可被分隔为前后两腔或左右两腔；②周围型粘连，粘连发生于两侧壁，宫腔狭小，两侧宫角可封闭，两侧壁内聚，严重的宫腔狭小呈桶状；③混合型，即合并有中央型和周围型两类粘连。

目前国际上采用最多的是美国生育协会的分类（表 7-1）。欧洲妇科内镜学会分类见表 7-2，中国宫腔粘连诊断分级标准见表 7-3。

表 7-1　美国生育协会评分标准

评估项目	项目标准描述	评分/分
粘连范围	<1/3	1
	1/3～2/3	2
	>2/3	4

续表

评估项目	项目标准描述	评分/分
粘连性质	菲薄	1
	部分菲薄部分致密	2
	致密	4
月经状态	无改变	0
	减少	2
	闭经	4

注：轻度或Ⅰ级，总分1～4分；中度或Ⅱ级，总分5～8分；重度或Ⅲ级，总分8～12分。

表7-2　欧洲妇科内镜学会分类

分度	项目标准描述
Ⅰ度	子宫腔内多处有纤维膜样粘连带，两侧宫角及输卵管开口正常
Ⅱ度	子宫前后壁间有致密的纤维粘连带，两侧宫角及输卵管开口可见
Ⅲ度	纤维索状粘连致部分宫腔及一侧宫角闭锁
Ⅳ度	纤维索状粘连致部分宫腔及两侧宫角闭锁
ⅤA	粘连带瘢痕化致宫腔极度变形及狭窄
ⅤB	粘连带瘢痕化致宫腔完全消失

表7-3　中国宫腔粘连诊断分级评分标准

评估项目	项目标准描述	评分/分
粘连范围	<1/3	1
	1/3～2/3	2
	>2/3	4
粘连性质	膜性	1
	纤维性	2
	肌性	4
输卵管开口状态	单侧开口不可见	1
	双侧开口不可见	2
	桶状宫腔，双侧宫角消失	4

续表

评估项目	项目标准描述	评分/分
子宫内膜厚度 （增殖晚期）	≥7 mm	1
	4~6 mm	2
	≤3 mm	4
月经状态	经量≤1/2 平时量	1
	点滴状	2
	闭经	4
既往妊娠史	自然流产 1 次	1
	复发性流产	2
	不孕	4
既往刮宫史	人工流产	1
	妊娠早期清宫	2
	妊娠中晚期清宫	4

注：轻度，总分 0~8 分；中度，总分 9~18 分；重度，总分 19~28 分。

二、治疗

1. 手术指征：有生育要求且有月经过少甚至闭经、不孕、反复流产等，或出现周期性腹痛、宫腔积血等症状者。

2. 麻醉选择：可酌情选择静脉麻醉、硬膜外或区域阻滞麻醉、全身麻醉。

3. 手术时机：手术前建议行 2~3 周期内膜准备，雌激素补充及扩血管治疗。月经干净 3~7 天，闭经则随时手术。

4. 术前准备：

（1）术前晚放置宫颈扩张棒扩张宫颈或阴道后穹隆放置米索前列醇 0.4 mg（排除米索前列醇禁忌证）软化宫颈，也可以术前静脉注射间苯三酚软化宫颈。

（2）对于近期做了宫腔镜检查或者分离术者，需要警惕已经发生了不全或者完全子宫穿孔的可能，对于可疑者，建议不要在 1 个月内再次行宫腔镜手术。

5. 手术操作流程：

（1）患者取膀胱截石位，用扩宫条逐步扩张宫口至大于镜体外鞘直径半号。接通液体膨宫泵，调整压力至 100 mmHg（13.3kPa），排空灌流管内气体，边膨宫边将宫腔镜置入宫腔。

（2）从远至近观察宫腔整体形态，宫腔的情况，宫腔内粘连的部位、范围及粘连性质类型，特别是宫底是否可见，输卵管开口是否可见。

（3）依据粘连类型、粘连范围酌情选择分离方法。膜性粘连及纤维性粘连可以用微型钳或微型剪撑开或剪开分离粘连；肌性粘连多以针状电极线型电切分离。

（4）术中要分清子宫腔的解剖学形态，操作时应根据中心对称原则，沿宫腔中线向两侧进行，以粘连疏松处作为突破口，撑开或者切开宫腔内粘连。有明显瘢痕形成的患者需要剔除或者剪除纤维瘢痕组织，直至当宫腔镜退至宫腔下段接近宫颈内口时，宫底部、双侧宫角显露及双侧输卵管开口可见，尽量恢复宫腔解剖学形态。若宫角致密粘连，不强求分离，以免发生术中穿孔及未来妊娠破裂，只要有足够宫腔，适时行体外受精－胚胎移植术（in vitro fertilization and embryo transfer，IVF-ET）。

6. 术中术后注意事项：

（1）分离粘连过程中特别强调手术中对正常子宫内膜的保护。对于膜性或纤维性粘连，采用微型剪刀或者微型钳撑开分离，当肌性瘢痕性粘连，需要使用能源电极时，用能分离粘连最低的电切频率，同时尽量使用针状电极减少能源电极与子宫内膜的接触面积，环状电极剔除瘢痕组织，暴露瘢痕下方的内膜组织，同时尽量缩短手术时间，减少内膜的热损伤。

（2）分离术中注意子宫腔的对称性。宫角和双输卵管开口是重要解剖标志。术前三维或四维超声，或者超声造影检查，术中可根据粘连程度酌情选用B超和（或）腹腔镜监护，都有利于宫角和输卵管开口的寻找。如术中无法看到典型的输卵管开口且不能确定分离层次时不要盲目分离。

（3）术中如果误入子宫肌层则可以清晰地看到粉红色和网格状的结构，同时可以看到明显的小血管，发现这些特征提示分离层次错误，需要及时停止手术，避免进一步发生子宫穿孔、宫壁假道、子宫出血等并发症，手术困难者不勉强进行，可分次手术。

（4）术中注意控制手术时间及膨宫液入量，预防水中毒的发生。粘连严重的患者，手术困难，手术时间长，术中血窦开放，容易出现液体吸收过多，发生水中毒。术中要尽量降低膨宫压力，将手术时间控制在半小时以内，将液体出入量的差值控制在 1000 mL 以内。如手术时间超过半小时，液体出入量差

>1000 mL，需要及时使用呋塞米 20 mg，若发生 TURP，呋塞米使用量不应超过 40 mg。

（5）术后宫腔隔离可选择放置宫腔用交联透明质酸钠、球囊或者羊膜制品防止宫腔再粘连。①放置球囊时，根据宫腔大小注入生理盐水 3~4 mL 形成球囊于宫腔，以不掉出为原则，同时避免球囊压力过高，压迫内膜导致缺血，5~7 天后取出。②使用羊膜时，将 2 片羊膜制品放入 25 ℃~30 ℃生理盐水中浸泡 15~20 分钟，使其适当复水展开，将其分别包裹于 Foley 球囊表面待用。再次扩张子宫颈管至 Hegar 扩张棒 10 号，抽吸 Foley 球囊内的液体或气体使球囊呈负压状，沿扩张的子宫颈管轻轻置入宫腔，由球囊导管注入 8~10 mL 生理盐水膨胀球囊并使羊膜制品充分贴附于宫腔创面，停滞 1~2 分钟后回抽球囊内液体使之留存 3~4 mL 阻隔宫腔创面，球囊导管外接引流袋留置 7 天，常规抗生素预防感染。术后 7 天取出球囊。

（6）雌激素或雌孕激素序贯促子宫内膜再生治疗：术后给予雌激素（2~4 mg/d）促子宫内膜修复治疗。或雌－孕激素序贯疗法，月经第 5 天开始使用戊酸雌二醇 2~4 mg/d，连续用药 21 天，21 天中的最后 6~10 天加用孕激素（如黄体酮胶丸 200 mg/d 或者地屈孕酮片 10 mg/d），注意关注雌激素应用的禁忌证和随访其副作用。

（7）营养内膜、改善子宫微循环治疗：用维生素 E、维生素 C、麒麟丸营养子宫内膜，阿司匹林改善子宫微循环，有 Meta 分析结果显示，宫腔粘连分离术（transcervical resection of adhesions，TCRA）术后辅以皮下注射生长激素（growth hormne，GH）可促进子宫内膜生长，改善月经状况及降低术后宫腔再粘连发生的风险。

（8）再次评估治疗效果：术后 1 个月再次宫腔镜检查，了解宫腔粘连治疗的效果，再次粘连或残留粘连者再次行粘连分离。对于月经恢复较理想者 3 个月后停药。术后 1、3、6、12 个月门诊随诊，了解月经恢复及子宫内膜情况。

（9）术后受孕方式的选择：轻度宫腔粘连和中度宫腔粘连内膜和宫腔恢复好者，宫腔镜二探时可同时行双侧输卵管插管通水检查输卵管通畅情况。如未合并子宫以外的原因和男方等不孕因素时，可尝试自然受孕。重度宫腔粘连患者，特别是复发者，可考虑辅助生殖技术治疗。

7. 诊治流程（图 7-1）：

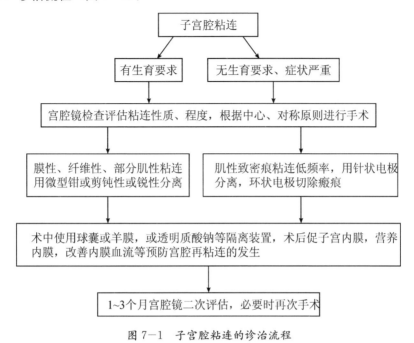

图 7-1　子宫腔粘连的诊治流程

李雪英　刘秋红

【参考文献】

［1］中华医学会妇产科学医学分会. 宫腔粘连临床诊疗中国专家共识［J］. 中华妇产科杂志，2015，50（12）：881-887.

［2］王欣，段华. 羊膜制品在重度宫腔粘连治疗中的应用及疗效分析［J］. 中华妇产科杂志，2016，51（1）：27-30.

［3］管媚媚，陈勃等. 宫腔镜下宫腔粘连分离术后预防再粘连方法比较［J］. 实用妇产科杂志，2016，32（7）：551-553.

［4］黄晓武. 宫腔镜下宫腔粘连分离术术中监护方法及操作要点［J］. 重庆医科大学学报，2017，42（4）：460-462.

［5］陈坤菊，史小荣，代晓琴. 宫腔粘连的预防方法研究进展［J］. 国际妇产科学杂志，2017，44（5）：576-580.

［6］李艳慧，邓荣，严凰群. 生长激素应用于宫腔粘连分离术后疗效的 Meta 分析［J］. 生殖医学杂志，2022，31（2）：233-239.

［7］FENG Q，GAO B，HUANG H，et al. Growth hormone promotes human endometrial glandular cells proliferation and motion through the GHR-STAT3/5 pathway［J］. Ann Transl Med，2020，8：53.

［8］BURJOOA，ZHAO X，ZOU L，et al. The role if preoperative 3D-ultrasound in intraoperative judgement for hysteroscopic adhesiolysis［J］. Ann Transl Med，2020，8（4）：55.

［9］向小珍，胡兵，李欢，等. 超声诊断宫腔粘连临床应用进展［J］. 中国介入影像与治疗学，2021，18（10）：631－634.

第八章　宫腔镜下输卵管
插管通液术手术操作规范

输卵管性不孕是输卵管粘连闭锁狭窄，影响受精卵通过导致的不孕，占女性不孕的 25%～35%，是女性不孕最主要的病因之一。引起不孕的输卵管病变包括输卵管近端梗阻、远端梗阻、全程阻塞、输卵管周围炎、输卵管功能异常和先天性输卵管畸形。输卵管性不孕的高危因素包括盆腔炎性疾病、异位妊娠史、盆腹部手术史、阑尾炎、宫腔操作史、子宫内膜异位症。既往检查输卵管是否通畅的方法有输卵管通水及输卵管造影。1998 年由 Gordts 首次采用经阴道注水腹腔镜-宫腔镜联合检查术用于诊治不孕症患者，借助生理盐水为膨胀介质，将内镜经阴道后穹隆置入盆腔，观察不孕症妇女盆腔解剖学结构并推求输卵管卵巢病变的微创诊断方法。因其视野范围仅可观察到盆腔的后半部分，难以检查出子宫前方的病变，有一定的漏诊率，且穿刺有一定的失败率，严重的盆腔粘连、子宫后倾固定及肥胖等易致穿刺失败和直肠穿孔。因此，对于经阴道注水腹腔检查的诊断准确性尚存在一定争议。近年来兴起的宫腔镜下输卵管插管通液术为输卵管不孕的治疗提供了新方法。

一、优点

1. 宫腔镜下输卵管插管通液术既能检查输卵管通畅情况，又能疏通或治疗输卵管阻塞。在直视下查找输卵管口，插入导管可机械扩张输卵管口，可去掉填塞输卵管口的血块、组织碎屑等；能明确地分侧进行输卵管通液，了解输卵管通畅情况，可使管腔内流体静压力增高，加上药液机械的冲刷作用，对输卵管起到扩张、利于消除炎症及疏通粘连的作用，可诊治近端输卵管阻塞。

2. 宫腔镜检查对宫腔的观察直观、清晰，是诊断宫腔病变的金标准，对于子宫输卵管造影（HSG）难以发现的粘连、息肉等一目了然，及时治疗，又避免了黏液、气泡等造成的误诊，还能发现引起不孕和反复流产的子宫异常或其他病变。

二、缺点

1. 需要操作者足够熟练，如插管方向不对，可能造成假阳性。

2. 其不能确定阻塞部位和输卵管形态，无法疏通输卵管远端的阻塞。

三、手术时间的选择

最佳时间在月经干净 3~7 天进行，过早月经未净，经血倒流，易导致子宫内膜异位；过迟内膜过长，输卵管口过小或不易发现，造成假梗阻，影响结果。

四、宫腔镜下输卵管插管通液治疗输卵管通畅程度的判断标准

1. 输卵管通畅：注入亚甲蓝无阻力、无反流，或有阻力但经适度加压、注液后阻力消失者为通畅。

2. 输卵管通而不畅：有一定阻力，适当加压推注后阻力下降，宫腔内亚甲蓝有少量反流。

3. 输卵管阻塞：推注阻力大，注液 8~10 mL 即不能再推注液体，宫腔内亚甲蓝反流多。

五、手术操作规范

取膀胱截石位，予 0.5％聚维酮碘消毒外阴、阴道及宫颈。静脉麻醉或经 1％利多卡因宫颈局部注射麻醉，置入宫腔镜，自宫颈管起检查宫颈内口状态，自远及近检查宫腔整体形态，若有异常可进一步检查局部情况，且逐渐深入宫底，检查两侧宫角及输卵管开口情况，调整开口处至视野中央，置入输卵管导管，自输卵管开口插入至输卵管间质部内深度≤1.5 cm，将稀释的亚甲蓝注入管腔内10 mL。根据推注阻力大小及是否存在液体往宫腔内反流现象，确定输卵管通畅度。并行超声监测输卵管有无异常膨胀及子宫直肠窝内有无积液。对输卵管

阻塞者改用小号注射器反复注水，以提高施加在输卵管腔内的压力，从而起到分离输卵管管腔内粘连的目的，继而注入药液（地塞米松、庆大霉素等混合液）进行通液治疗。

六、手术操作技巧

1. 插管时避免在输卵管口周围反复插戳，引起子宫收缩，输卵管口闭合，造成假梗阻。

2. 插管时还应注意插入的角度与输卵管间质部行经方向尽量保持同轴。

3. 推注液体时，一开始力量应由小逐渐加大，避免突然用力造成输卵管痉挛或破裂。

七、术后注意事项

术后给予口服抗生素预防感染，并禁止性生活2周。

张建平

【参考文献】

[1] 林小娜，黄国宁，孙海翔，等. 输卵管性不孕诊治的中国专家共识 [J]. 生殖医学杂志，2018，27（11）：1048－1056.

[2] 陈瑶，李曼丽，徐根儿，等. 影响宫腔镜下输卵管插管通液术治疗输卵管性不孕疗效的多因素分析 [J]. 中国微创外科杂志，2010，10（11）：1026－1028.

[3] 徐根儿，陈瑶. 宫腔镜输卵管插管通液术在输卵管性不孕诊治中的应用 [J]. 中国微创外科杂志，2013，13（05）：436－438.

[4] 张凌云，张保萍，方进芬，等. 宫腔镜下输卵管插管通液术在输卵管性不孕症治疗中的临床应用分析 [J]. 中国实用医药，2014（24）：74－75.

[5] 赵菊芬，杨柳风，李茜，等. 经阴道注水腹腔镜－宫腔镜联合检查与标准腹腔镜检查在不孕症中的临床评价 [J]. 中国妇幼保健，2016，31（4）：876－878.

[6] 廖会姝. 122例输卵管性不孕症的临床情况及宫腹腔镜下输卵管插管介入治疗的应用分析 [J]. 中国性科学，2020，29（2）：68－71.

第九章 子宫内膜非典型增生和早期子宫内膜样癌保留生育功能诊治流程及手术操作规范

　　子宫内膜非典型增生及子宫内膜样癌的病因，多与长期无孕激素拮抗的雌激素暴露有关。约30％的子宫内膜非典型增生患者会进展为子宫内膜样癌。对于无生育要求的子宫内膜非典型增生和子宫内膜样癌患者，首选手术治疗。而保留生育功能治疗仅适用于有强烈保留生育功能愿望，能坚持随访，并经严格选择的子宫内膜非典型增生及早期（Ⅰa期，G1）子宫内膜样癌患者。

一、诊断

　　1. 临床表现：育龄妇女可表现为不规则子宫出血、月经周期延长或缩短、出血时间长、出血量时多时少，有时表现为经间出血，月经周期规则但经期长或经量过多。绝经后妇女出现阴道出血是子宫内膜癌的主要症状，有90％以上绝经后子宫内膜癌患者有阴道出血症状。其他症状：包括阴道异常排液、宫腔积液、下腹疼痛等。

　　2. 体格检查：早期患者体格检查多无异常发现。

　　3. 影像学检查：经阴道超声可了解子宫大小、宫腔形状、宫腔内有无赘生物、子宫内膜厚度、肌层有无浸润及深度，可对异常阴道流血的原因做出初步判断，并为选择进一步检查提供参考。子宫内膜增生多表现为内膜厚，回声不均匀，局部可呈团块状。典型子宫内膜癌的超声图像有宫腔内不均回声区，或宫腔线消失、肌层内有不均回声区。彩色多普勒可显示丰富血流信号。磁共振成像对肌层浸润深度和宫颈间质浸润有较准确的判断，盆腹腔增强磁共振或增强CT可协助判断有无子宫外转移。

4. 诊断性刮宫：是常用的且有价值的诊断方法。常行分段诊刮以同时了解宫腔和宫颈的情况。对病灶较小者，诊断性刮宫可能会漏诊。组织学检查是确诊依据。

5. 宫腔镜检查：可直接观察宫腔及宫颈内有无癌灶存在，癌灶大小及部位，直视下活检，对局灶型子宫内膜癌的诊断和评估宫颈是否受侵更为准确。但不能判断侵犯肌层情况，宫腔镜是否将肿瘤细胞冲入腹腔影响预后目前依据不足。

6. 子宫内膜微量组织学或细胞学检查：操作方法简便，国外文献报道其诊断的准确性与诊断性刮宫相当。

7. 糖类抗原 125（CA125）测定：有子宫外转移或浆液性癌，血清 CA125 值可升高。

二、鉴别诊断

1. 子宫黏膜下肌瘤或内膜息肉：有月经过多或不规则阴道流血，可行超声检查、宫腔镜检查以及诊断性刮宫以明确诊断。

2. 内生型子宫颈癌、子宫肉瘤及输卵管癌：均可有阴道排液增多或不规则出血。内生型子宫颈癌因癌灶位于宫颈管内，宫颈管变粗、硬或呈桶状。子宫肉瘤可有子宫明显增大、质软。输卵管癌以阴道流血、下腹隐痛、间歇性阴道排液为主要症状，可有附件包块。分段诊刮及影像学检查可协助鉴别。

三、治疗

1. 保留生育功能的适应证：

（1）诊刮后病理诊断为子宫内膜非典型增生，或子宫内膜样癌Ⅰa期、G1，并经病理专家会诊核实。

（2）有强烈保留生育功能的要求。

（3）年龄为 40 岁及以下，最大不超过 45 岁。

（4）子宫内膜样癌病灶局限于子宫，影像学检查（最好 MRI）无肌层浸润、附件累及或远处转移证据。

（5）无药物治疗或妊娠禁忌。

（6）有良好依从性、随访条件，能再次行子宫内膜病理检查。

但因子宫内膜癌是手术病理分期，因此，以上各种评估方法都存在一定的局限性。

2. 宫腔镜手术评估适应证：

（1）盲刮病理确诊为子宫内膜非典型增生和早期子宫内膜样癌（子宫内膜样癌Ⅰa期、G1）有强烈保留生育功能要求的患者。

（2）保留生育功能治疗期间，每3~6个月进行宫腔镜下宫腔及子宫内膜的全面评估，对子宫内膜进行精准活检，去除病灶。

3. 麻醉选择：静脉麻醉或者宫颈管黏膜表面麻醉。

4. 手术时机：盲刮病理确诊后；保留生育功能治疗3~6个月后。

5. 术前准备：

（1）病情告知与知情选择：对于已确诊为子宫内膜非典型增生和早期子宫内膜样癌（子宫内膜样癌Ⅰa期、G1），但要求保留生育功能的患者，应告知患者，保留生育功能并非子宫内膜非典型增生和早期子宫内膜样癌的标准治疗方式，详细告知保留生育功能治疗可能存在的风险，包括治疗无效、治疗期间进展缓慢及完全缓解后复发的可能，并签署知情同意书。

（2）宫颈准备：术前晚酌情宫颈备管或采用高分子亲水宫颈扩张棒。

（3）术前禁食6小时以上。

6. 宫腔镜子宫内膜病灶切除术操作流程：

（1）取膀胱截石位，静脉麻醉后，常规消毒铺巾，探查宫颈深度后，扩张宫颈至7号，生理盐水作为膨宫介质，接通液体膨宫泵，调整压力值100 mmHg（13.3kPa），排空灌流管内气体，边膨宫边缓慢置入宫腔镜。

（2）宫腔镜下按顺序仔细检查宫颈、宫底和子宫前、后、左、右壁，以及双侧宫角和子宫下段近颈管处，详细记载宫腔形态、深度，黏膜颜色、厚度等，并详细记录病变部位、大小、形态、范围等，有条件的医院可采用窄带成像技术（narrow-band imaging，NBI）检查并可保留宫腔镜图片及影像学资料。

（3）根据宫腔镜检查对可疑病变使用微型钳钳夹病变部位组织，对背景子宫内膜随机取样或搔刮取样。

（4）对病变组织行子宫内膜病灶电切术：膨宫压维持在70~80 mmHg（9.3~10.7kPa）；充分扩张宫颈至10号扩宫棒顺利进入，置入10 mm电切镜，5 mm切割环，调整输出功率至280 W；使用电切环一般切除深度可以达到肌层表面，但不要切除肌层，对于高度怀疑子宫内膜癌变的患者使用垂直电切环切开子宫底部，将病灶及子宫浅肌层 3 mm（大约一个电切环的深度）切除，病灶组织术中送检。

（5）切除病灶后对子宫增压，以观察是否存在病灶残留；确保病灶完全清除后，降低宫压，若无出血等不良症状则排出膨宫液。

7. 术中术后注意事项：

（1）掌握阳性病灶典型镜下表现：①内膜厚度不均，可有局部隆起或新生物，呈结节性、乳头状或息肉状的隆起，表面灰白或有白点状或斑状组织；②腺体开口排列重度不规整或消失，伴有钙化、坏死；③可见异型血管，表现为血管中断、扩张、狭窄、曲折、屈曲、锯齿状。其中，具有中心血管的半透明绒毛状突起群，呈海葵状，很可能是子宫内膜高分化腺癌的特征性表现。

（2）术中注意正常内膜的保护，切忌遍刮宫腔，电切病灶时降低电切频率，避免能源电极对周围内膜组织的电损伤，预防电切术后的子宫腔粘连，保护患者生育功能。

（3）低膨宫压力，缩短操作时间，避免膨宫压力增加而出现肿瘤细胞向腹腔扩散。

（4）保留生育功能的患者术后需结合其他综合治疗方案，术后一般是每 3 个月宫腔镜评估宫腔情况 1 次，直至病变逆转（连续两次评估呈阴性）。

8. 诊治流程（图 9-1）：

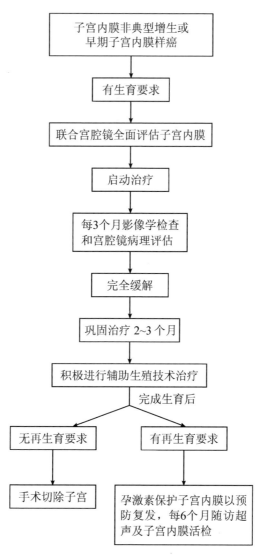

图 9-1 子宫内膜非典型增生和早期子宫内膜癌的诊治流程

卢艳　唐溪瞳

【参考文献】

[1] 陈晓军，杨佳欣，王英华，等. 子宫内膜非典型增生和早期子宫内膜样癌保留生育功能治疗及评估的建议 [J]. 中华妇产科杂志，2019，54（2）：80－86.

[2] 王永学，潘凌亚，黄慧芳，等. 年轻子宫内膜癌患者孕激素保守治疗临

床分析 [J]. 中华肿瘤学防治杂志，2011，18（7）：541－544.

[3] 曹冬焱，俞梅，杨佳欣，等. 大剂量孕激素治疗早期子宫内膜癌及子宫内膜不典型增生患者的妊娠结局及相关因素分析 [J]. 中华妇产科杂志，2013，48（7）：519－522.

[4] 俞梅，杨佳欣，曹冬焱，等. 早期子宫内膜癌保留生育功能治疗后复发的诊治 [J]. 山东大学学报（医学版），2018，56（5）：23－29.

[5] 何翙姣，王益勤，汤惠如，等. 子宫内膜非典型增生及早期子宫内膜癌复发后再次保留生育功能治疗的临床疗效及妊娠结局 [J]. 中华妇产科杂志，2020，55（1）：21－28.

[6] 全国卫生产业企业管理协会妇幼健康产业分会生殖内分泌学组. 中国子宫内膜增生诊疗共识 [J]. 生殖医学杂志，2017，26（10）：957－959.

[7] Francesca Falcone，Giuseppe Laurelli，Simona Losito，et al. Fertility preserving treatment with hysteroscopic resection followed by progestin therapy in young women with early endometrial cancer [J]. J Gynecol Oncol，2017，28（1）：e2.

[8] Paolo Casadio，Francesca Guasina，Roberto Paradis，et al. Fertility-sparing treatment of endometrial cancer with initial infiltration of myometrium by resectoscopic surgery：a pilot study [J]. Oncologist，2018，23（4）：478－480.

[9] 陈娇，孔为民，宋丹，等. 宫腔镜检查对Ⅱ型子宫内膜癌患者腹腔细胞学结果及预后的影响 [J]. 现代妇产科进展，2016，25（4）：257－260.

第十章　应用 PDCA 循环
减少宫腔镜术中 TURP 综合征发生率

经前列腺电切综合征（transurethral resection of prostate syndrome，TURP syndrome），简称 TURP 综合征，又称水中毒。如诊治不及时可致死亡，是宫腔镜手术中的严重并发症之一，是由于膨宫压力较高、子宫内膜及肌层血管床破坏较广、手术时间较长等多种原因导致的灌流介质过多进入人体，造成体液超负荷和（或）稀释性低钠血症（指采用非生理盐水膨宫介质时）从而引起的一系列临床症状。

不同的灌流介质引起的症状不同。单极能源系统灌注介质主要是低渗的、低黏度的非电解质溶液，包括 5％葡萄糖、5％甘露醇、3％山梨醇、1.5％甘氨酸，双极电能源要求使用电解质溶液（生理盐水、乳酸林格液）。目前，临床应用最多的灌注介质为生理盐水。非电解质灌流液进入循环后，很快经肝脏代谢生成多量水分，导致血浆离子浓度降低，血浆的总体渗透压下降，进而引起脑水肿；如不能及时纠正，可能导致永久性脑损伤，甚至死亡。电解质液体中的离子可以维持血浆的总体渗透压水平，在一定限度内即使有过量的液体吸收，患者也极少出现低钠血症。此外，不同的灌流介质其代谢产物不同，可能引起一些相应的临床表现，1.5％甘氨酸可引起高氨血症、一过性视物模糊，山梨醇可诱发高钙血症，5％葡萄糖可能引起血糖升高等。尽管应用生理盐水灌流很少发生低钠血症，但有高氯性酸中毒的报道。

一、理由

1. 手术并发症的发生率是国家三级公立医院绩效考核重要指标之一，也是三甲医院评审的重要指标之一。

2. 笔者所在科室宫腔镜三级、四级手术占比高，手术难度大，手术并发症风险高。TURP 综合征是宫腔镜手术的严重并发症，一旦出现可导致 15%～40% 的死亡率。

为了降低 TURP 综合征发生率，成立持续质量改进（continous quality improvement，CQI）小组，成员情况如表 10-1 所示。

表 10-1　CQI 小组成员

序号	姓名	职称	组内职务	职责分工
1	李雪英	主任医师	组长	组织、学习手术并发症管理
2	张建平	主任医师	副组长	协调、组织、实施手术
3	卢艳	主任医师	副组长	组织管理病人、实施手术
4	刘秋红	副主任医师	组员	组织管理病人、实施手术
5	杨丽娟	副主任医师	组员	组织管理病人、实施手术
6	陈亮	主任医师	组员	监管全科麻醉师职责培训
7	覃芳	副主任护士	组员	监管手术室护士的职责培训

二、现状调查

2021 年 1—4 月，笔者所在的科室宫腔镜手术共 632 例，对发生 TURP 综合征的病例进行回顾性统计分析，如图 10-1 所示。

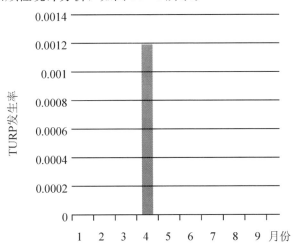

图 10-1　2021 年 1—4 月宫腔镜术中 TURP 综合征发生率

根据图 10-1 分析，笔者所在科室 2021 年 1—4 月宫腔镜手术发生 TURP 综合征共 2 例，均发生在 4 月份，2 例均进入 ICU 治疗。根据以上数据分析，必须采取有效措施控制 TURP 综合征发生率，才能更好地提高我们手术质量，更好地为患者保驾护航。

三、目标确定

TURP 综合征的发生率是多种因素引起，为了规避这些因素导致 TURP 综合征的发生率，笔者所在的科室成立了由科主任、副主任医师、麻醉师、手术室护士长共同组成 CQI 手术质量安全小组。经讨论分析拟定如何将宫腔镜发生 TURP 综合征的发生率在 2021 年 1—9 月份 2 例的基础上降低，以后尽量保持无宫腔镜发生 TURP 综合征。

四、原因分析

2021 年 1—9 月宫腔镜手术 2 例宫腔镜术中术后发生水中毒病例，总结分析发生 TURP 综合征原因，运用头脑风暴法进行讨论，分析笔者所在的科室宫腔镜手术发生 TURP 综合征并发症的原因如图 10-2 所示。

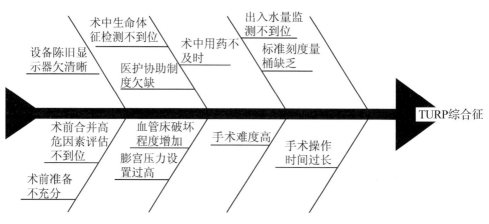

图 10-2　发生 TURP 综合征并发症的原因

五、要因确认

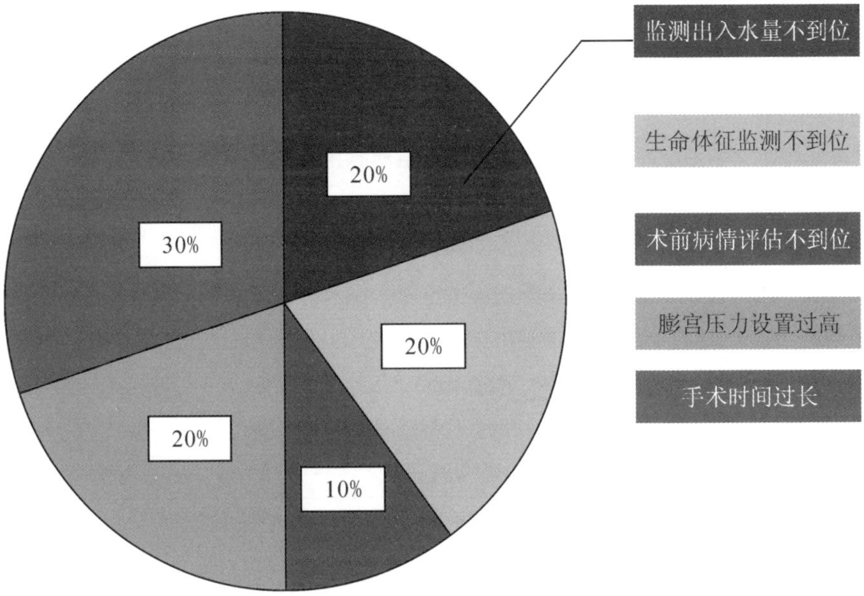

图 10-3 宫腔镜手术发生 TURP 综合征主要因素分析图

六、制订对策

TURP 综合征对策见表 10-2。

表 10-2 TURP 综合征对策

序号	主要原因	计划与措施	责任人	计划完成时间
1	监测出入水量不到位，工作责任感不强	加强手术室医护职责制度学习，执行不到位者，严肃批评教育并与绩效挂钩。 完善手术室内相关配套物品（备标准出水桶），对于陈旧设备及时报备，审批更换。	覃芳	2021 年 5 月 10 日
2	监测生命体征不到位	加强医护职责制度学习，执行不到位者，严肃批评教育并与绩效挂钩。	陈亮	2021 年 5 月 10 日

续表

序号	主要原因	计划与措施	责任人	计划完成时间
3	术前病情评估不到位，术前合并高危因素未引起重视	对于年龄偏大、贫血患者术前应充分进行风险评估，及时纠正贫血，减少手术风险。	刘秋红	2021年5月
4	术中膨宫压力选择	尽量选择低于平均动脉压膨宫压力，压力通常选用80～100 mmHg（10.7～13.3kPa）为宜	卢艳 刘秋红	2021年5月
5	手术时间过长	术中根据具体情况，手术时间尽量控制在60分钟以内，出入水量差值不超过2500 mL。对于难度大、一次性不能完成手术者，选择二次手术完成。	卢艳 刘秋红	2021年5月

七、对策实施

1. 组织学习宫腔镜并发症相关知识，正确认识TURP综合征。

2. 认真学习宫腔镜预防TURP综合征相关措施，形成TURP综合征处理流程。

3. 手术室麻醉师及巡回护士加强18项核心制度学习，增加手术室标准出水桶的用量。

4. 制作TURP综合征处理流程图（图10-4）。

5. 制订预防TURP综合征具体措施：①术前纠正贫血等高危因素；②术中严密观察生命体征；③降低膨宫压力至100～120 mmHg（13.3～16.0 kPa）；④尽量控制手术操作时间在60分钟内；⑤术中使用宫缩剂减少血窦开放、减少灌流液吸收，呋塞米利尿减轻血容量负荷；⑥严格计算出入量，控制出入水量差值在2500 mL以内；⑦大的肌瘤必要时预处理或分期手术。

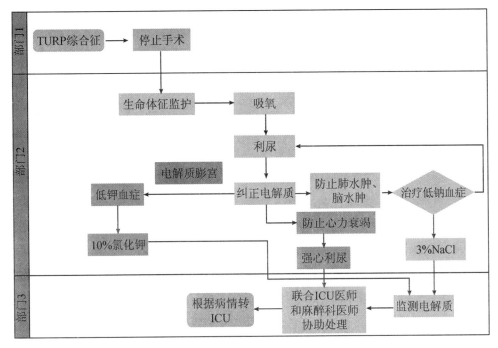

图 10-4　TURP 综合征处理流程图

八、效果评价

2021 年 1—4 月，笔者科室宫腔镜手术共 632 例，TURP 综合征的发生率为 0.31%，5—9 月宫内疾病与介入中心住院宫腔镜手术累计共 528 台，其中宫腔镜发生 TURP 综合征 0 例，TURP 综合征发生率明显降低。

九、巩固措施

1. 邀请专家授课及指导，学习相关 TURP 综合征的防治措施。
2. 组织人员外出进修或参加短期培训班培训。
3. 定期对医务人员进行 TURP 综合征防治的考核。
4. 每例 TURP 综合征并发症科室都会总结分析，提出持续改进措施。

十、下一步计划

为进一步提高医疗质量与安全，科内将进一步提升医务人员的理论水平及业务工作能力，进一步加强宫腔镜并发症的质量监控，通过"PDCA"循环改进，减少宫腔镜其他并发症发生率。

瞿慧　李雪英

【参考文献】

［1］黄晓武，夏恩兰. 解读宫腔镜手术并发症：TURP 综合征［J］. 国际妇产科学杂志，2014，41（5）：566－569，574.

［2］张颖，段华，张师前. 2020 年美国妇产科医师学会和美国妇科腔镜医师协会《子宫腔内病变的宫腔镜诊治专家共识》解读［J］. 中国实用妇科与产科杂志，2020，36（9）：907－910.

第十一章　宫腔镜手术护理常规

宫腔镜手术是应用膨宫介质扩张宫腔，通过导光玻璃纤维束和柱状透镜将冷光源经宫腔镜导入宫腔内，在直视下观察宫颈管、宫颈内口、子宫内膜和输卵管开口，能够直接观察宫腔内的生理与病理变化，可针对病变组织直接取材送病检，并在直视下进行宫腔内手术治疗。

一、护理常规

1. 按一般妇科护理常规。

2. 术前护理：

（1）检查时间一般以月经干净后 3～7 天内为宜。

（2）术前完善各项体格检查和辅助检查：门诊手术患者行血常规、尿常规、凝血功能、输血四项、白带常规、细菌性阴道病（BV）、心电图、宫颈液基薄层细胞（TCT）、人乳头瘤病毒（HPV）监测等检查，必要时行支原体、衣原体、淋病奈瑟菌等检查。住院手术患者需要加做 X 线胸片、肝肾功能、血型等检测，必要时行泌尿系超声等检查。

（3）监测血压、脉搏、体温，术前禁食 6～8 小时，禁饮禁水 2 小时。

（4）入手术室前取下义齿、首饰，佩戴口罩，同时排空膀胱。

（5）与手术室工作人员交接：

1）核对患者基本信息：病历（病室、床号、姓名、性别、年龄、诊断）及手腕带标识。

2）交接患者情况：生命体征、手术名称、各类导管（输液管、导尿管、引流管等）通畅否、皮肤等情况。

3）交接特别医嘱、输入液体药物和液体输注情况，以及所携带的特殊物品和药品，是否取下义齿、首饰等。

3. 术后护理：

（1）与手术室工作人员交接：

1）核对患者基本信息：床头卡、病历（病室、床号、姓名、性别、年龄、诊断）及手腕带标识。

2）交接患者情况：生命体征、麻醉方式、手术名称、各类导管（输液管、导尿管、引流管等）通畅否、皮肤等情况。

3）交接特别医嘱、输入液体药物和液体输注情况，以及所携带的特殊物品和药品等。

（2）测量生命体征并记录，有异常及时向医生汇报。

（3）体位：不限制，患者感觉舒适即可。

（4）早活动：麻醉清醒后患者即可根据自己的活动能力下床活动，首次下床活动需注意预防跌倒/坠床的发生。

（5）饮食护理：术后无恶心等特殊不适，即可进营养丰富的软食，减少刺激性食物的摄入。

（6）观察排尿情况，有排尿困难者先诱导排尿，必要时遵医嘱给予导尿。

（7）观察阴道流血情况：

1）手术创面大、出血多的患者，多在术中放置宫腔水囊管压迫止血，术后观察引流袋内血量，一般每天小于 20 mL，最多不超过 50 mL。如引流袋内血量小于 10 mL，术后 24～48 小时内拔除宫腔水囊管。如 24 小时引流袋内血量大于50 mL 应该及时报告医生。

2）注意观察阴道出血情况，如术后阴道流血多于月经量，应及时报告医生，遵医嘱给予处理。

（8）留置宫腔水囊管的护理：

1）维持良好的固定，引流管低于会阴口，妥善安全放置。

2）保持引流管通畅，防止管道扭曲、移位、堵塞、脱落或受压。指导患者保持大便通畅。

3）观察引流袋内引流液的颜色、性状、量，每天更换引流袋。

4）注意外阴卫生，遵医嘱药液擦洗会阴，每天 2 次，预防感染。

5）一般留置时间不超过 2 周。

（9）疼痛的护理：

1）评估患者疼痛程度。

2）提供安静舒适的环境，分散患者注意力。嘱患者放松，多可自行缓解。

3）必要时遵医嘱给予镇痛药物，并观察用药后效果。

二、健康指导

1. 手术后健康宣教：向患者及陪伴家属讲解宫腔镜术后注意事项，以配合护理工作。

2. 指导患者保持个人清洁卫生。

3. 性生活指导：术后禁性生活及盆浴 1 个月。

4. 术后休息 1 个月，避免体力劳动。

林波

【参考文献】

［1］谢幸，孔北华，段涛. 妇产科学 .［M］. 9 版. 北京：人民卫生出版社，2018：435－437.

［2］Practice guidelines for moderate procedural sedation and analgesia 2018：a report by the american society of anesthesiologists task force on moderate procedural sedation and analgesia，the American association of oral and maxillofacial surgeons，American college of radiology，American dental association，American society of dentist anesthesiologists，and society of interventional radiology. Anesthesiology，2018，128（3）：437－479.

［3］中国心胸血管麻醉学会日间手术麻醉分会. 宫腔镜诊疗麻醉管理的专家共识［J］. 临床麻醉学杂志，2020，36（11）：1121－1125.

［4］杨万玲，徐秀萍. 快速康复外科护理在门诊宫腔镜围手术期中的应用［J］. 临床护理杂志，2014，13（2）：42－44.

附　录

附录A　《宫腔镜在宫内疾病诊治中的应用》
2020 美国妇产科医师学会专家共识解读

2020 年 3 月，由美国妇产科学会（American College of Obstetricians and Gynecologists，ACOG）与美国妇科腹腔镜医师协会（American Association of Gynecological Laparoscopists，AAGL）共同发表了用以替代 2018 年 9 月 ACOG 公布的《宫腔镜技术评价》。随着宫腔镜的普及，大量宫腔镜检查及手术在门诊施术。这个专家共识关注了门诊宫腔镜的基本设施、患者选择、术者要求、相关疼痛管理及后续随访问题。第一次提出阴道内镜的操作方法，尤其应该应用于门诊宫腔镜的诊断与治疗。同时，本共识更注重宫腔镜检查及手术中特有的并发症的高危因素探讨，及时诊断和积极治疗。本文对新版专家共识进行简要的介绍及讨论。

一、宫腔镜检查的一般注意事项

应用宫腔镜诊断技术要熟知膨宫介质的管理、最佳诊断时机和宫颈准备。

1. 膨宫介质：膨宫是为了在宫腔镜手术中获得足够的视野。以往使用 CO_2 和高黏度膨宫介质，如右旋糖酐等已不再推荐。有关低黏度灌流液的特点见附表 A-1，特别提出最大负欠量的标准。有关更多细节，请参阅 AAGL 宫腔镜膨宫介质管理实践指南[1]。

附表 A-1　宫腔镜低黏度膨宫介质

类型	最大液体负欠量	优点	缺点	并发症
非电解质溶液（1.5% 甘氨酸；3% 山梨醇；5% 葡萄糖和 5% 甘露醇）	1000 mL	单极和射频能量兼容	过度吸收可导致稀释性低钠血症	过度吸收会导致低钠血症、高氨血症和血浆渗透压降低，可能导致癫痫发作、脑水肿和死亡
电解质溶液（如生理盐水，乳酸钠溶液）	2500 mL	便于获取等张液体诊断性宫腔镜检查和使用机械、激光或双极能量的手术中可选择的介质	尽管使用这些介质可以减少低钠血症和血浆渗透压降低的风险，但肺水肿和充血性心力衰竭仍然可能发生	液体超负荷导致肺水肿和充血性心力衰竭

2. 检查时机：月经周期正常者诊断宫腔镜的最佳时机是在月经后的卵泡期，检查前必须先排除妊娠。在分泌期检查增厚的子宫内膜可能会与息肉相混淆，增加诊断困难。月经不规律者可以随时安排宫腔镜检查，但出血多不建议手术，术野可能受限。孕激素或口服避孕药的预处理可以使子宫内膜变薄，改善视野清晰度、缩短手术时间。虽然促性腺激素释放激素（gonadotropin-releasing hormone，GnRH）激动剂的预处理也能薄化子宫内膜、减少出血、降低黏膜下肌瘤去除术难度，但由于其不良反应，常规并不推荐，仅在严重贫血患者中，GnRH-α 有利于手术前的预处理和提高血红蛋白水平[2]。

3. 宫颈软化：没有足够的证据建议在宫腔镜诊断或探查术前常规促宫颈成熟，仅对宫颈狭窄或手术增加疼痛风险较高的患者可以考虑。需要平衡宫颈软化的潜在益处与药物不良反应之间的关系[3]。宫颈软化常用方法包括舌下含服、口服或阴道用前列腺素，如米索前列醇；物理扩张法如阴道一次性扩张棒。手术前4 小时阴道内给药 400 μg 米索前列醇已被证明可以减少门诊宫腔镜中和检查后的疼痛，可能是因为减少了没必要的宫颈扩张。研究证实，在手术前 14 天阴道用 25 μg 雌激素，以及在手术前 12 小时阴道置 400～1000 μg 米索前列醇，对于绝经后患者更容易宫颈扩张和减轻疼痛[4,5]。但在中国的药品说明书上米索前列醇仅用于妊娠期终止妊娠，请中国医生特别知晓。渗透性扩张剂与米索前列醇的比较，同样减少了扩宫的操作，但增加了额外操作，如果患者由于其他原因没有接受本次手术，扩张器又不得不再次取出。

在局部麻醉剂中加入稀释的血管收缩剂，如加压素或肾上腺素，以帮助宫颈扩张。其潜在益处包括减少出血和减少液体过吸收，增加麻醉的持续时间和麻醉效力，以及减少全身吸收和局部麻醉剂的毒性，但建议谨慎使用这些药物，特别是在门诊宫腔镜中，因为有可能发生罕见但严重的心血管事件，包括心动过缓、低血压或高血压和心脏骤停。

二、宫腔镜手术

使用手术宫腔镜可治疗子宫内膜息肉、子宫肌瘤、子宫纵隔、妊娠残留物和粘连等宫内疾患。手术宫腔镜的其他适应证包括清除异物，如嵌顿的宫内节育器、输卵管插管，治疗宫颈管阻塞和定位活检。

息肉去除术推荐的手术方法包括宫腔镜直视下使用剪刀和抓钳等冷刀去除术、单极或双极能源性去除术，或宫腔镜下刨削系统的去除术。对于多发息肉去除术，宫腔镜下直视去除优先于盲刮手术，这与刮宫手术的高漏诊率相关。

子宫肌瘤的宫腔镜手术指征是异常子宫出血、反复流产和不孕症，其手术并发症发生率为 $1\% \sim 5\%$ [6]。宫腔镜下肌瘤切除术的成功取决于黏膜下肌瘤的类型（尤其是肌层穿透程度）。

在随机试验中，宫腔镜下肌瘤切除过程中使用稀释加压素溶液可显著减少术中失血和扩张液吸收[7,8]。目前尚不清楚 GnRH-α 能否作为常规宫腔镜下肌瘤切除术前辅助药物，这需要更多高质量的数据来支持术前使用 GnRH-α 能够减少手术时间、灌流液吸收和重复手术的次数。

宫腔镜下肌瘤切除能否一次性完成主要取决于平滑肌瘤的特点。肌瘤多个、直径大、侵犯肌层深，或者肌瘤对侧同时有需要去除的肌瘤，可能需要分步手术，以实现完全的手术切除，同时尽量减少宫内粘连的形成[9,10]，肌瘤未能一次性切除的主要因素为灌流液过吸收。

三、宫腔镜下手术组织病理的获取方式

传统宫腔电切镜使用单极或双极环将切除组织碎片经宫颈取出，通常需要反

复进入宫腔，对宫颈和宫腔可能造成医源性损伤。新的宫腔镜下组织去除系统（刨削系统）已经问世，在组织切除同时将标本取出。刨削系统优点是手术时间较短，与传统的电切镜相比，完全切除病变（子宫内膜息肉、0型或Ⅰ型肌瘤）的可能性较高[11,12]。其缺点包括一次性设备及其特有的膨宫系统的成本较高；在某些类型的刨削设备中缺乏电外科器械，无法电凝止血；因刨削系统无法有效分离Ⅱ型平滑肌瘤的包膜，去除这类肌瘤的能力有限。

四、门诊宫腔镜的特殊注意事项

许多诊断性宫腔镜和手术性宫腔镜正在从手术室转移到门诊施术。在随机研究中，与住院手术宫腔镜相比，患者更倾向于门诊宫腔镜，门诊宫腔镜有更高的患者满意度，患者康复也更快。其他潜在好处包括对患者和医生来说更为便捷，避免全身麻醉，熟悉的门诊环境能够减少患者焦虑，卫生经济学效益更佳，更有效地将复杂的宫腔镜手术让位于住院手术处理。

该技术首要适应证是子宫内膜息肉。门诊宫腔镜下息肉切除术已被证明是安全的，具有良好的耐受性，与传统的住院宫腔镜息肉去除术相比更具成本效益。在多中心随机试验中，结果表明随访12个月和24个月门诊手术治疗异常子宫出血的病例数不亚于住院手术。

五、患者咨询和选择

门诊宫腔镜的应用必须建立有效的异常子宫出血的诊断评估流程。能否选择门诊宫腔镜手术取决于对疾病的良恶性判断、病变大小、病变穿透深度、患者是否愿意接受门诊手术、医生技能和专门知识、对患者并发症的评估、合适的设备和器械，以及对患者的关爱。例如，某些患有合并症的患者，如睡眠呼吸暂停或心肺疾病，在没有麻醉护理的情况下，可能不适合进行门诊静脉镇静。对于那些焦虑或既往门诊宫腔镜失败或不耐受门诊施术的患者，应该考虑在另一种环境下进行宫腔镜检查，如手术室或门诊手术中心。

六、阴道内镜检查方法

阴道内镜是一种手术技术，不使用阴道窥器和宫颈抓钳，置入宫腔镜以显示阴道、宫颈、宫腔结构。外径纤细的宫腔镜可用作阴道内镜。阴道内镜技术包括将宫腔镜置入阴道，多使用生理盐水为膨宫介质以扩张阴道。与传统的宫腔镜相比，阴道内镜检查方法可以大大减少术中疼痛。此外，将阴道内镜技术与传统宫腔镜进行比较时，手术的失败率无显著性差异。ACOG 和 AAGL 都建议门诊宫腔镜检查时可以考虑应用阴道内镜的手术方法。

可以通过夹闭大小阴唇的方法避免灌流液自阴道内泄漏。宫腔镜进入阴道后直接进到后穹隆，旋转宫腔镜光纤识别宫颈外口。宫腔镜进入宫颈管内，顺应子宫前屈或后屈位置缓慢进入子宫腔。如果子宫过度前倾可以在耻骨联合上方施压或充盈膀胱减少子宫屈度，如果子宫过度后屈可以通过直肠指诊前压减少子宫后屈。

七、疼痛管理

文献中常用的门诊宫腔镜镇痛方案包括单一的药物或多种药物的组合，包括局部麻醉剂、非甾体抗炎药、对乙酰氨基酚、苯二氮䓬类、阿片类，也可选择宫颈内或宫颈旁阻滞，或两者兼而有之。根据目前已有证据，与安慰剂相比，这些方法在疼痛管理的安全性或有效性方面没有临床意义上的差异。有研究证实宫旁阻滞可以减少宫腔镜通过宫颈时的疼痛[13]。许多研究证实门诊宫腔镜患者可以耐受，可不使用任何镇痛，如果先前存在疼痛状况，如痛经或慢性盆腔疼痛时可能需使用镇痛治疗。目前没有一个单一的方案或一组药物被证明在临床上优于安慰剂。

八、门诊宫腔镜的设置

在实施门诊宫腔镜手术时，必须优先考虑患者的安全性和舒适性。安全性保障包括在门诊设置更多的信息提示、与患者及其家属有效沟通、工作人员专业能力、防范药物的错误使用、周密的患者随访机制和常规流程的可行性。

门诊宫腔镜检查应在适当空间、设备和人员配置的治疗室进行。基本设置要求包括宫腔镜设备、摄像机和显示器、膨宫系统以及清洁和消毒设备。没有足够的证据建议优先使用某种特定类型的宫腔镜，宫腔镜的选择应由操作者自行决定。

九、并发症的预防和管理

最大的两项多中心研究分别为 13 600 例诊断和手术宫腔镜及 21 676 例手术

宫腔镜，总并发症率分别为 0.28％和 0.22％[14,15]。潜在并发症的发生率及危险因素见附表 A-2。

附表 A-2　宫腔镜手术潜在并发症、发生率及高危因素

潜在并发症	发生率	高危因素
穿孔	0.12％~1.61％	盲目置入器械，宫颈狭窄，解剖结构改变（如平滑肌瘤和先天性异常，宫腔内粘连，子宫内膜菲薄，子宫极端前倾或后倾）
空气和气体栓塞	0.03％~0.09％	反复进入宫腔，膨宫管流入道内有气体，宫内压力过大
流体超负荷	0.20％	过度吸收任何灌流液，切除的病灶大，侵犯深肌层和宫内高压；使用非电解质灌流液增加低钠血症的风险，以及脑水肿
出血	0.03％~0.61％	宫颈裂伤，子宫穿孔，粘连松解，宫内病变切除
迷走神经反射	0.21％~1.85％	牵拉宫颈和进行宫颈管内及宫腔内操作时触发宫旁副交感神经

1. 穿孔：最常见的围手术期并发症是子宫穿孔，其处理取决于穿孔的位置、原因和严重程度。宫腔镜手术的每一步骤，包括机械性宫颈扩张、探测宫腔、宫腔镜置入、使用电外科器械或刨削装置，都可能导致子宫肌层损伤。虽然缺乏宫腔镜检查中假道发生率的数据，但这种并发症很可能发生在进入宫腔及其困难的病例中，这可能增加子宫穿孔的风险。穿孔造成大出血、可疑内脏损伤，或电外科电极穿孔需要立即手术探查。

2. 感染：抗生素预防不推荐用于常规宫腔镜手术。在盆腔感染活动期和活动期疱疹感染时禁止进行宫腔镜检查。对 1 952 例手术宫腔镜的前瞻性观察研究中，粘连松解后子宫内膜炎的风险高于平滑肌瘤或息肉切除术[16]。在随机研究中诊断或手术宫腔镜后，抗生素预防尚未被证明能减少术后感染。

3. 电外科损伤：电外科能源产生的严重损伤可发生在宫腔镜手术中，尤其伴发于子宫穿孔时。如果出现明显的内出血或怀疑内脏器官有热损伤，应该即刻进行探查。下生殖道（如阴道或会阴）也可能有热损伤的风险。潜在的危险因素包括宫

颈过度扩张，器械绝缘层缺损，或激活电极时外鞘没有在宫颈管内进行充分保护。

4. 液体超负荷：灌流液过度吸收可导致严重的并发症，包括肺水肿、神经系统并发症和死亡。使用非电解质、低渗膨宫介质造成低渗低钠血症和脑水肿的风险更大。通过缜密的围手术期计划，使用先进的灌流系统和评估要去除的宫腔内病变，可以减少灌流液的超负荷。灌流液的超负荷与切除病变的大小和数目、肌层侵犯深度、肌层血窦开放程度和宫内压力密切相关。灌流液监测指南如下：

（1）宫腔镜手术围手术期应密切监测血电解质变化，术中应密切监测宫腔镜灌流液吸收情况。

（2）对于老年患者、合并症患者、心血管或肾脏损害患者，以及遇到急诊状况抢救能力有限的地方，应考虑降低灌流液过吸收的阈值。

（3）在健康患者中，低渗溶液的最大负欠量为 1 000 mL，等渗溶液为 2 500 mL。如果负欠量达到 750 mL 低渗溶液、2 000 mL 等渗溶液则应考虑停止手术，并与麻醉人员共同讨论处理方案。

（4）在急救和化验检测有限的门诊环境中，应考虑降低灌流液负欠量的阈值，及时停止手术。

（5）一个自动化实时监测系统有助于尽早发现灌流液的过吸收。

（6）应指定专人检测出入量，并随时向术者报告。

（7）如果出现超过阈值，尤其是低渗溶液，需评估患者的血液动力学、神经系统、呼吸和心血管状态以及评估液体过吸收的特有症状和体征。应检测血清电解质和渗透压，考虑使用利尿剂，并根据化验指标进行诊断和治疗干预。静脉注射呋塞米有助于利尿，15~20 分钟后临床症状改善。进一步治疗液体超负荷或低钠血症可能需要使用高渗液体，须专家指导诊疗，必要时转至 ICU。

5. 空气和气体栓塞：空气或气体栓塞来源可能是作为宫腔镜膨宫介质的 CO_2，进入子宫颈或子宫腔的室内空气，单极或双极激发时产生的气体，或在最初截石位摆放时进入的空气。气体的化学性质影响栓塞的风险。CO_2 在血液中的溶解度高于氧气；因此，来自房间空气（含氧气和氮气）的空气栓塞的风险大于 CO_2 气体栓塞的风险[17]。空气或气体栓塞的严重性包括心脏/肺衰竭或死亡。空气或气体栓塞的最常见症状为呼吸困难和胸痛，呼末 CO_2 压力降低或血流动力学状态改变（低血压、心动过速）时应该引起临床上对栓塞的怀疑。听诊大水轮音（"磨轮"杂音）是一个经典的体征，尽管其不是在所有情况下都被检测到。

预防方法包括从宫腔镜灌流液注入道和器械通道中尽可能排出空气；尽量减少反复进入宫腔，因为这可能会以"活塞样"的方式将空气带入子宫；消除宫内气泡；限制宫内压力。急性空气和气体栓塞的治疗包括迅速停止手术、回抽宫腔内气体和消除气体来源。采用 Durant 急救法，患者左侧卧位和头低脚高位时可以促进空气或气体向右心室的迁移，以减少右心室流出道处的阻塞。

6. 出血：对于出血的管理，可以采用各种止血措施，这取决于出血的严重程度、性质和出血位置；但关于这些技术的有效性数据不足。止血方法包括电凝术、使用宫内球囊（Foley 导管）、子宫动脉栓塞、注射加压素或肾上腺素、氨甲环酸和子宫切除术。

7. 血管迷走神经反射：一旦发现迷走神经反射（低血压、心动过缓）或症状（恶心、呕吐、多汗、面色苍白或意识丧失），应停止手术，并进行患者评估和抢救（生命体征，包括脉搏、血压和"ABC"——气道、呼吸和循环支持）。大多数迷走神经反射可通过变换体位解决，如抬高患者的腿或呈头低脚高位。如果症状或心动过缓持续存在，可给予阿托品。

孙宇婷　冯力民

【参考文献】

［1］MUNRO M G，STORZ K，ABBOTT J A，et al. AAGL practice report：practice guidelines for the management of hysteroscopic distending media：（replaces hysteroscopic fluid monitoring guidelines. J Am Assoc Gynecol Laparosc. 2000；7：167－168.）AAGL Advancing Minimally Invasive Gynecology Worldwide. ［J］J Minim Invasive Gynecol，2013，20（2）：137－148.

［2］KAMATH M S，KALAMPOKAS E E，KALAMPOKAS T E. Use of GnRH analogues pre-operatively for hysteroscopic resection of submucous fibroids：a systematic review and meta-analysis ［J］. Eur J Obstet Gynecol Reprod Biol，2014，177：11－18.

［3］GKROZOU F，KOLIOPULOS G，VREKOUSSIS T，et al. A systematic review and meta-analysis of randomized studies comparing misoprostol versus placebo for cervical ripening prior to hysteroscopy ［J］. Eur J Obstet Gynecol Reprod Biol，2011，158（1）：17－23.

［4］CASADE L，PICCOLO E，MANICUTI C，et al. Role of vaginal estradiol pretreatment combined with vaginal misoprostol for cervical ripening before operative hysteroscopy in postmenopausal women ［J］. Obstet Gynecol Sci，2016，59（3）：220－226.

［5］OPPEGAARD K S，LIENG M，BERG A，et al. A combination of misoprostol and estradiol for preoperative cervical ripening in postmenopausal women：a randomised controlled trial ［J］. BJOG，2010，117（1）：53－61.

［6］Alternatives to hysterectomy in the management of leiomyomas. ACOG Practice Bulletin No. 96. American College of Obstetricians and Gynecologists ［J］. Obstet Gynecol，2008，112：387－400.

［7］PHILLIPS D R，NATHANSON H G，MILIM S J，et al. The effect of dilute vasopressin solution on the force needed for cervical dilatation：a randomized controlled trial ［J］. Obstet Gynecol，1997，89（4）：507－511.

［8］WONG A S，CHEUNG C W，YEUNG S W，et al. Transcervical intralesional vasopressin injection compared with placebo in hysteroscopic myomectomy：a randomized controlled trial ［J］. Obstet Gynecol ，2014，124（5）：897－903.

［9］TASKIN O，SADIK S，ONOGLU A，et al. Role of endometrial suppression on the frequency of intrauterine adhesions after resectoscopic surgery ［J］. J Am Assoc Gynecol Laparosc，2000，7（3）：351－354.

［10］YANG J H，CHEN M J，WU M Y，et al. Office hysteroscopic early lysis of intrauterine adhesion after transcervical resection of multiple apposing submucous myomas ［J］. Fertil Steril，2008，89（5）：1254－1259.

［11］SMITH P P，MIDDLETON L J，CONNOR M，et al. Hysteroscopic morcellation compared with electrical resection of endometrial polyps：a randomized controlled trial ［J］. Obstet Gynecol，2014，123（4）：745－751.

［12］LI C，DAI Z，GONG Y，et al. A systematic review and meta-analysis of randomized controlled trials comparing hysteroscopic morcellation with resectoscopy for patients with endometrial lesions ［J］. Int J Gynaecol Obstet，2017，136（1）：6－12.

[13] KANESHIRO B, GRIMES D A, LOPES L M. Pain management for tubal sterilization by hysteroscopy [J]. Cochrane Database of Systematic Reviews, 2012, (8): CD009251.

[14] JANSEN F W, VREDEVOOGD C B, VAN ULZEN K, et al. Complications of hysteroscopy: a prospective, multicenter study [J]. Obstet Gynecol, 2000, 96 (2): 266−270.

[15] AYDENIZ B, GRUBER I V, SCHAUF B, et al. A multicenter survey of complications associated with 21,676 operative hysteroscopies [J]. Eur J Obstet Gynecol Reprod Biol, 2002, 104 (2): 160−164.

[16] AGOSTINI A, CRAVELLO L, SHOJAI R, et al. Postoperative infection and surgical hysteroscopy [J]. Fertil Steril, 2002, 77 (4): 766−768.

[17] GROENMAN F A, PETERS L W, RADEMAKER B M, et al. Embolism of air and gas in hysteroscopic procedures: pathophysiology and implication for daily practice [J]. J Minim Invasive Gynecol, 2008, 15 (2): 241−247.

The Use of Hysteroscopy for the
Diagnosis and Treatment of Intrauterine Pathology

ABSTRACT: This Committee Opinion provides guidance on the current uses of hysteroscopy in the office and the operating room for the diagnosis and treatment of intrauterine pathology and the potential associated complications. General considerations for the use of diagnostic and operative hysteroscopy include managing distending media, timing for optimal visualization, and cervical preparations. In premenopausal women with regular menstrual cycles, the optimal timing for diagnostic hysteroscopy is during the follicular phase of the menstrual cycle after menstruation. Pregnancy should be reasonably excluded before performing hysteroscopy. There is insufficient evidence to recommend routine cervical ripening before diagnostic or operative hysteroscopy, but it may be considered for those patients at higher risk of cervical stenosis or increased pain with the surgical procedure. In randomized trials, patients reported a preference for office-based hysteroscopy, and office-based procedures are associated with higher patient satisfaction and faster recovery when compared with hospital-based operative hysteroscopy. Other potential benefits of office hysteroscopy include patient and physician convenience, avoidance of general anesthesia, less patient anxiety related to familiarity with the office setting, cost effectiveness, and more efficient use of the operating room for more complex hysteroscopic cases. Appropriate patient selection for office-based hysteroscopic procedures for women with known uterine pathology relies on thorough knowledge and understanding of the target pathology, size of the lesion, depth of penetration of the lesion, patient willingness to undergo an office-based procedure, physician skills and expertise, assessment of patient comorbidities, and availability of proper equipment and patient support. Both the American College of Obstetricians and Gynecologists (ACOG) and the American Association of Gynecologic Laparoscopists (AAGL) agree that vaginoscopy may be considered when performing office hysteroscopy because studies have shown that it can significantly reduce procedural pain with similar efficacy. The office hysteroscopy analgesia regimens commonly described in the literature include a single agent or a combination of multiple agents, including a topical anesthetic, a nonsteroidal antiinflammatory drug, acetaminophen, a benzodiazepine, an opiate, and an intracervical or paracervical block, or both. Based on the currently available evidence, there is no clinically significant difference in safety or effectiveness of these regimens for pain management when compared to each other or placebo. Patient safety and comfort must be prioritized when performing office hysteroscopic procedures. Patients have the right to expect the same level of patient safety as is present in the hospital or ambulatory surgery setting.

Recommendations and Conclusions

The American College of Obstetricians and Gynecologists and the American Association of Gynecologic Laparoscopists (AAGL) make the following conclusions and recommendations regarding the use of hysteroscopy for the diagnosis and treatment of intrauterine pathology:

- In premenopausal women with regular menstrual cycles, the optimal timing for diagnostic hysteroscopy is during the follicular phase of the menstrual cycle after menstruation. Pregnancy should be reasonably excluded before performing hysteroscopy.

- Some women with unpredictable menses can be scheduled at any time for operative hysteroscopy, but ideally patients who are actively bleeding may not undergo the procedure because adequate visualization could be impaired.

- There is insufficient evidence to recommend routine cervical ripening before diagnostic or operative hysteroscopy, but it may be considered for those patients at higher risk of cervical stenosis or increased pain with the surgical procedure.

- Intravaginal misoprostol administration of 400 micrograms has been shown to decrease pain during and after office hysteroscopy when administered at least 4 hours before the procedure, likely because of the decreased need for dilation. Data support that with the addition of 25 micrograms vaginal estrogen 14 days before the procedure, along with $400 - 1000$ micrograms vaginal misoprostol 12 hours before the procedure, ease of cervical dilation and reduction in pain was substantial in postmenopausal patients.

- Potential advantages of hysteroscopic tissue removal systems are shorter operative time and higher likelihood of complete lesion removal (endometrial polyp, type 0 or I leiomyoma) compared with conventional resectoscopy. Potential disadvantages of these systems include the cost of the disposable devices along with their associated fluid management systems; the lack of electrosurgical element in some of these types of devices, resulting in the inability to cauterize bleeding vessels; and limited data on the capability to treat type II leiomyomas.

- In randomized trials, patients reported a preference for office-based hysteroscopy, and office-based procedures are associated with higher patient satisfaction and faster recovery. Other potential benefits of office hysteroscopy include patient and physician convenience, avoidance of general anesthesia, less patient anxiety related to familiarity with the office setting, cost effectiveness, and more efficient use of the operating room for more complex hysteroscopic cases.

• Office hysteroscopy for the treatment of endometrial polyps should be considered whenever possible.

• Appropriate patient selection for office-based hysteroscopic procedures for women with known uterine pathology relies on thorough knowledge and understanding of the target pathology, size of the lesion, depth of penetration of the lesion, patient willingness to undergo an office-based procedure, physician skills and expertise, assessment of patient comorbidities, and availability of proper equipment and patient support.

• Vaginoscopy may be considered when performing office hysteroscopy because studies have shown that it can significantly reduce procedural pain with similar efficacy.

• The office hysteroscopy analgesia regimens commonly described in the literature include a single agent or a combination of multiple agents, including a topical anesthetic, a nonsteroidal antiinflammatory drug, acetaminophen, a benzodiazepine, an opiate, and an intracervical or paracervical block, or both. Based on the currently available evidence, there is no clinically significant difference in safety or effectiveness of these regimens for pain management when compared to each other or placebo.

• Antibiotic prophylaxis is not recommended for routine hysteroscopic procedures.

• Complications from fluid overload may be minimized with careful perioperative planning, use of a fluid management system, and evaluation of the intracavitary lesions to be removed.

This Committee Opinion provides guidance on the current uses of hysteroscopy in the office and the operating room for the diagnosis and treatment of intrauterine pathology and the potential associated complications.

General Considerations for the Use of Hysteroscopy

General considerations for the use of diagnostic and operative hysteroscopy include managing distending media, timing for optimal visualization, and cervical preparations. Obstetrician-gynecologists should be familiar with these principles.

Distending Media

The uterus requires distention for adequate visualization of the cavity during hysteroscopy. Historically, carbon dioxide gas and high-viscosity fluid media such as dextran were used. See Table 1 for information on the potential advantages, disadvantages, and complications of currently used hysteroscopic distending media, as well as guidance on maximum fluid deficit. For additional details, see *AAGL Practice Report: Practice Guidelines for the Management of Hysteroscopic Distending Media*[1].

Optimization of Visualization

In premenopausal women with regular menstrual cycles, the optimal timing for diagnostic hysteroscopy is during the follicular phase of the menstrual cycle after menstruation. Pregnancy should be reasonably excluded before performing hysteroscopy. Hysteroscopy during the secretory phase of the cycle may make diagnosis more difficult because a thickened endometrium may mimic polyps. Some women with unpredictable menses can be scheduled at any time for operative hysteroscopy, but ideally patients who are actively bleeding may not undergo the procedure because adequate visualization could be impaired. Pretreatment with progestins or combined oral contraceptives may improve visualization by thinning the endometrium[2-4]. Data support that pretreatment with combination oral contraceptives may improve visualization at the time of polypectomy and increase surgical satisfaction compared with timed procedures, even with short courses of therapy[3]. Although pretreatment with gonadotropin-releasing hormone (GnRH) agonists also thins the endometrium and may reduce blood loss and improve visualization with submucous myomectomy, they are not routinely recommended because of adverse effects; however, in patients with severe anemia, they are beneficial for surgical preparation and optimizing hemoglobin levels before surgery[5].

Table 1. Hysteroscopic Distending Media

Type	Maximum Fluid Deficit	Advantages	Disadvantages and Safety Precautions *	Complications
Low-Viscosity Fluid Media: Electrolyte-Poor Fluid (eg, glycine, 1.5%; sorbitol, 3%; and mannitol, 5%)	1,000 mL	Compatible with radiofrequency energy Monopolar devices require electrolytepoor fluids	Excessive absorption of these fluids can cause hyponatremia, hyperammonemia, and decreased serum osmolality with the potential for seizures, cerebral edema, and death.	Excessive absorption of these fluids can lead to hyponatremia, hyperammonemia, and decreased serum osmolality, with the potential for seizures, cerebral edema, and death.
Low-Viscosity Fluid Media: Electrolyte-Containing Fluid (eg, normal saline, sodium lactated solution)	Maximum fluid deficits with isotonic solutions are based only on expert opinion but consensus would be approximately 2,500 mL.	Readily available Isotonic Media of choice during diagnostic hysteroscopy and in operative cases where mechanical, laser, or bipolar energy is used	Although the risk of hyponatremia and decreased serum osmolality can be reduced by using these media, pulmonary edema and congestive heart failure can still occur. Careful attention should be paid to fluid input and output, with particular attention to the fluid deficit.	Fluid overload causing pulmonary edema and congestive heart failure

* Careful attention should be paid to fluid input and output, with particular attention to the fluid deficit, particularly in elderly patients and patients with cardiopulmonary or renal compromise, in whom lower fluid thresholds should be considered.

Data from Munro MG, Storz K, Abbott JA, Falcone T, Jacobs VR, Muzii L, et al. AAGL practice report: practice guidelines for the management of hysteroscopic distending media: (replaces hysteroscopic fluid monitoring guidelines. J Am Assoc Gynecol Laparosc, 2000, 7: 167 −168). AAGL Advancing Minimally Invasive Gynecology Worldwide. J Minim Invasive Gynecol, 2013, 20: 137−148.

Preoperative Ripening of the Cervix

There is insufficient evidence to recommend routine cervical ripening before diagnostic or operative hysteroscopy, but it may be considered for those patients at higher risk of cervical stenosis or increased pain with the surgical procedure. The potential benefits should be weighed against the increased risk of adverse effects of the medication[6]. Options for cervical preparation methods include sublingual, oral, or vaginal prostaglandin, such as misoprostol; and vaginal osmotic dilators, such as laminaria. A 2015 systematic review concluded that use of misoprostol for preoperative ripening is more effective than placebo or no treatment and is associated with fewer intraoperative complications; however, it is associated with a higher rate of adverse effects, including mild abdominal pain, increased body temperature, and vaginal bleeding[7]. In women undergoing diagnostic hysteroscopy in the operating room or the office setting, misoprostol has been studied at various dosages, most frequently 200−400 micrograms orally or vaginally, and has demonstrated a decrease in procedural times, improved ease of cervical entry, and decreased pain scores[8, 9]. Intravaginal misoprostol administration of 400 micrograms has been shown to decrease pain during and after office hysteroscopy when administered at least 4 hours before the procedure, likely because of the decreased need for dilation[10]. Data support that with the addition of 25 micrograms vaginal estrogen 14 days before the procedure, along with 400−1000 micrograms vaginal misoprostol 12 hours before the procedure, ease of cervical dilation and reduction in pain was substantial in postmenopausal patients[11, 12]. In women undergoing operative hysteroscopy, misoprostol administration at various dosages and by different routes has been shown to decrease the need for mechanical dilation over placebo[7, 13]. A comparison of osmotic dilators versus misoprostol demonstrated a decreased need for mechanical dilation with a similar side effect profile for osmotic dilators; however, an additional office visit for osmotic dilator placement before hysteroscopy may make this a less desirable choice for patients and health care providers[6, 14]. Also, if the patient does not undergo surgery for any reason, the dilator will need to be removed.

Some clinicians may consider adding a vasoconstricting agent, such as vasopressin or epinephrine, to the local anesthetic to aid with cervical dilation. Potential benefits of vasoconstrictor use include reduction in procedural blood loss and fluid absorption, increase in the duration and potency of anesthesia, and decrease in systemic absorption and toxicity of the local anesthetic[15]. An additional cited advantage of intracervical dilute vasopressin is reduction in the force required for mechanical cervical dilation, although there is variability in dosage in practice. For example, a randomized, double-blind study of 52 women used 20 mL of a dilute solution (4 units of 0.05 units/mL of vasopressin in 80 mL of normal saline)[16]. Cautious administration of these agents is recommended, especially in the office setting, given the possibility of rare but serious cardiovascular events including bradycardia, hypotension or hypertension, and cardiac arrest[17, 18].

Operative Hysteroscopy

Obstetrician-gynecologists use operative hysteroscopy to treat intrauterine pathology such as endometrial polyps, uterine leiomyomas, uterine septa, retained products of pregnancy, and adhesions. Additional uses of operative hysteroscopy include the removal of foreign bodies such as malpositioned intrauterine devices, tubal cannulation, treatment of isthmoceles, and directed biopsy.

Hysteroscopic Polypectomy and Myomectomy

Indications for polyp removal include abnormal uterine bleeding, infertility, and recurrent pregnancy loss. Management of endometrial polyps consists of expectant management or surgical management, depending on patient symptoms and risk factors for malignancy within the endometrial polyp[19]. Surgical resection techniques that can be used involve blind polyp removal or curettage; direct visualization and removal using hysteroscopic scissors and grasping forceps, monopolar or bipolar resectoscopes; or hysteroscopic mechanical tissue removal devices. For polypectomy, direct hysteroscopic removal is preferred over blind procedures, which are associated with inaccurate detection and ineffective removal of intrauterine lesions[20, 21].

Hysteroscopic myomectomy is widely used for the treatment of abnormal uterine bleeding in the setting of submucosal uterine leiomyoma. Other specific indications for hysteroscopic removal of submucosal leiomyoma include recurrent pregnancy loss and infertility. The reported complication rate for hysteroscopic myomectomy ranges between 1% and 12%, with rates of 1−5% reported in most studies[22]. The success of hysteroscopic myomectomy is dependent on the type of submucosal leiomyoma (eg, the degree of myometrial penetration).

The use of dilute vasopressin solution during hysteroscopic myomectomy has been shown to decrease intraoperative blood loss and distention fluid absorption significantly in two randomized trials[16, 23]. The benefit of GnRH agonists as an adjunct before routine hysteroscopic myomectomy is unclear. More high-quality data are needed to support the use of preoperative GnRH agonists to reduce operative time, distending fluid absorption, and the need for repeat surgery.

Proper patient counseling regarding surgical outcomes and the ability to perform a single versus staged procedure is based upon leiomyoma characteristics. A two-step procedure may be required for patients with multiple, large, deep, or opposing leiomyomas to achieve complete surgical resection, minimize intrauterine adhesion formation, or both[24, 25]. A small observational study noted 70.2%, 54.8%, and 44.2% of patients were surgery-free at 1, 2, and 3 years respectively after incomplete hysteroscopic myomectomy for type Ⅱ leiomyomas. Mean age of this patient population was 42.5 years and the majority of these cases were terminated because of fluid absorption[26].

Hysteroscopic resection of endometrial polyps and submucosal leiomyomas can be performed using either monopolar or bipolar wire loop electrodes. Although the use of a monopolar resectoscope requires an electrolyte-free distending medium (eg, 1.5% glycine or 3% sorbitol), bipolar resectoscopes can be used with electrolyte-containing distending medium (eg, normal saline). Another less commonly used hysteroscopic surgical technique is electrosurgical vaporization, which uses a large surface-area vaporization electrode set at higher power density settings (eg, 120−220 watts) compared with the power density used for conventional wire loop electrodes. Vaporization devices allow for destruction of targeted lesions without the creation of tissue fragments, thereby eliminating the need for tissue removal; however, this also prohibits histologic evaluation of tissue, which may be necessary in some clinical scenarios. See Box 1 for additional types of intrauterine pathology that may be diagnosed and treated with hysteroscopy.

Box 1. Situations When Hysteroscopy May Be Used * △

• Removal of foreign bodies (eg, intrauterine devices with nonvisualized strings or intrauterine devices that are malpositioned)

• Diagnosis and treatment of intrauterine adhesions

• Correction of septate uteri

• Detection of malignancy

• Management of cesarean scar pregnancy

• Management of retained products of pregnancy or focal accreta

• Detection and treatment of isthmocele

• Tubal cannulation

* Excluding Endometrial Polyps and Leiomyoma

△Less common conditions managed by hysteroscope may require referral to a high-volume clinician or clinician with expertise in hysteroscopy.

Hysteroscopic Treatment of Intrauterine Pathology

Traditionally, targeted removal of intrauterine pathology using a monopolar or bipolar wire loop resectoscope required transcervical specimen removal of tissue fragments, often involving repetitive introduction of surgical instruments with potential for increased trauma to the cervix and uterus. Newer hysteroscopic tissue removal systems have emerged, allowing for the removal of lesions by simultaneous tissue resection and specimen extraction. Potential advantages of hysteroscopic tissue removal systems are shorter operative time and higher likelihood of complete lesion removal (endometrial polyp, type 0 or I leiomyoma) compared with conventional resectoscopy[27-29]. Potential disadvantages of these systems include the cost of the disposable devices along with their associated fluid management systems; the lack of electrosurgical element in some of these types of devices, resulting in the inability to cauterize bleeding vessels; and limited data on the capability to treat type Ⅱ leiomyomas[30]. Additionally, type Ⅱ leiomyomas may be more difficult to remove with these devices, compared to the loop resectoscope that could dissect the myoma from surrounding myometrium. Blind removal is not indicated where instrumentation for guided removal is available[21].

Special Considerations for Office Hysteroscopy

Many diagnostic hysteroscopy and operative hysteroscopy procedures are being shifted from the operating room to an office-based setting. In randomized trials, patients reported a preference for office-based hysteroscopy and office-based procedures are associated with higher patient satisfaction and faster recovery when compared with hospital-based operative hysteroscopy[31, 32]. Other potential benefits of office hysteroscopy include patient and physician convenience, avoidance of general anesthesia, less patient anxiety related to familiarity with the office setting, cost effectiveness, and more efficient use of the operating room for more complex hysteroscopic cases.

If the technology is available, office hysteroscopy for the treatment of endometrial polyps should be considered. Office hysteroscopic polypectomy has been shown to be safe, well tolerated, and more cost-effective compared with traditional inpatient hysteroscopic polypectomy[33]. In a multicenter randomized trial, outpatient polypectomy was found to be noninferior to inpatient polypectomy for the treatment of abnormal uterine bleeding, with similar treatment effects maintained at 12 months and 24 months[34]. Both a multicenter, randomized, controlled, noninferiority study and a multicenter, prospective observational trial found that office hysteroscopic polypectomy may be associated with a higher risk of failed or incomplete polyp removal[34,35]. Conversely, inpatient hysteroscopic polypectomy may be associated with greater risk of complications[34, 35].

Patient Counseling and Selection

The use of office hysteroscopy has been well established for the diagnostic evaluation of abnormal uterine bleeding[36]. Appropriate patient selection for office-based hysteroscopic procedures for women with known uterine pathology relies on thorough knowledge and understanding of the target pathology, size of the lesion, depth of penetration of the lesion, patient willingness to undergo an office-based procedure, physician skills and expertise, assessment of patient comorbidities, and availability of proper equipment and patient support. For example, patients with medical conditions, such as sleep apnea or cardiopulmonary disease, may not be appropriate candidates for office-based intravenous sedation without the presence of an anesthesia care team. Consideration for performing hysteroscopy in an alternative setting, such as the operating room or ambulatory surgery center, should be made for patients who have anxiety or have previously failed or not tolerated the office-based procedure.

Vaginoscopic Approach to Hysteroscopy

Vaginoscopy is a surgical technique involving the insertion of a hysteroscope to visualize the vagina, cervix, uterine cavity, or all of these structures, without the use of a vaginal speculum or cervical tenaculum. Small-diameter rigid or flexible hysteroscopes can be used as vaginoscopic instrumentation. A vaginoscopic technique involves gentle introduction of the hysteroscope into the vagina and use of distending medium, such as normal saline, to expand the vaginal canal. The vaginoscopic approach has been shown to reduce procedural pain substantially compared with traditional hysteroscopy. Furthermore, no significant difference was found in the number of failed procedures when comparing vaginoscopic technique with traditional hysteroscopy[37-40]. Both ACOG and AAGL agree that vaginoscopy may be considered when performing office hysteroscopy because studies have shown that it can significantly reduce procedural pain with similar efficacy[41].

Minimizing fluid leakage from the vagina can be accomplished by manual compression of the labial tissue to narrow the vaginal introitus. The hysteroscope is directed toward the posterior vaginal fornix and the external cervical os is identified. Guidance of the hysteroscope into the endocervical canal and subsequently into the uterine cavity is facilitated by knowledge of the uterine position and correction of anteflexion or retroflexion, if necessary. Techniques to bring the uterus into axial position include applying direct pressure above the pubic symphysis or full bladder distention to reduce uterine anteflexion, and placing anterior pressure digitally through the rectum to decrease uterine retroflexion[42].

Pain Management

The office hysteroscopy analgesia regimens commonly described in the literature include a single agent or a combination of multiple agents, including a topical anesthetic, a nonsteroidal antiinflammatory drug, acetaminophen, a benzodiazepine, an opiate, and an intracervical or paracervical block, or both. On the basis of the currently available evidence, there is no clinically significant difference in safety or effectiveness of these regimens for pain management when compared with each other or placebo[43]. Paracervical blocks have been shown to decrease pain at the time of tenaculum placement and passage of the hysteroscope through the external and internal os[44]. Other evidence has shown that office hysteroscopy may be tolerated without the use of any analgesia, although preexisting pain conditions such as dysmenorrhea or chronic pelvic pain may warrant its use[45]. No single regimen or group of medications has been shown to be clinically superior to placebo.

Office Preparation

Patient safety and comfort must be prioritized when performing office hysteroscopic procedures. Patients have the right to expect the same level of patient safety as is present in the hospital or ambulatory surgery setting[46]. See ACOG's *Report of the Presidential Task Force on Patient Safety in the Office Setting* for more information on effective communication, staff competency, medication error avoidance, accurate patient tracking mechanisms, anesthesia safety, and general procedural safety[46]. The use of procedure checklists, logs, and mock drills can promote consistent behavior and documentation to allow for quality review.

Office hysteroscopy should be performed in an appropriately sized, equipped, and staffed treatment room. Basic set-up requirements for in-office hysteroscopy include hysteroscopic instrumentation, camera and monitor, delivery system for distending media, and facilities to clean, disinfect, and sterilize equipment. There is insufficient evidence to recommend preferential use of a specific type of hysteroscope, and the choice of hysteroscope should be left to the discretion of the operator[41].

Cleaning of reusable hysteroscopic devices is necessary before disinfection or sterilization. Protocols for disinfection and sterilization of equipment may vary depending on the type of equipment used and should adhere to manufacturer's guidelines and comply with institutional, state, and federal regulations.

Prevention and Management of Complications

The two largest multicenter studies of 13,600 diagnostic and operative hysteroscopies and 21,676 operative hysteroscopies found overall complication rates of 0. 28% and 0. 22% respectively[47, 48]. Significantly more complications occurred during operative hysteroscopy than during diagnostic hysteroscopy (0. 95% versus 0. 13%; P, 0. 01). See Table 2 for potential complications, incidence, and risk factors.

Perforation

The most common perioperative complication of hysteroscopic surgery is uterine perforation[48, 49]. Known risk factors for uterine perforation are listed in Table 2. Management of uterine perforation is dependent on the location, cause, and severity of the uterine perforation. Each step of hysteroscopy, including mechanical cervical dilation, uterine sounding, hysteroscope insertion, or the use of electrosurgery or tissue removal device, may result in compromise of the uterine myometrium. Although data on the incidence of false passage creation during hysteroscopy are lacking, this complication may occur in cases of difficult uterine

Table 2. Potential Complications, Incidence, and Risk Factors of Hysteroscopy

Potential Complication	Incidence	Risk Factors
Perforation	0.12% to 1.61%[1][2][3]	Blind insertion of instruments, cervical stenosis, anatomic distortion (eg, leiomyomas and congenital anomalies, intrauterine adhesions, myometrial thinning, and uterine malposition [extreme anteversion or retroversion])
Air and gas embolism (clinically significant)	0.03% to 0.09%[4][5]	Repetitive instrumentation through cervix, inadequate purging of air from tubing and instruments, excessive intrauterine pressure
Fluid overload	0.20%[2]	Excessive absorption of any distending fluid, resection of large or deep lesions and high intrauterine pressure; increased risk of hyponatremia with use of electrolyte-free distending media, and cerebral edema with hypotonic distending media.
Hemorrhage	0.03% to 0.61%[1][2][6]	Cervical laceration, uterine perforation, adhesiolysis, resection of cavitary lesions
Vasovagal reaction	0.21% to 1.85%[7]	Triggering of parasympathetic nervous system during manipulation of the cervix and instrumentation of the cervical canal or uterine cavity

①AYDENIZ B, GRUBER I V, SCHAUF B, KUREK R, MEYER A, WALLWIENER D. A multicenter survey of complications associated with 21,676 operative hysteroscopies. Eur J Obstet Gynecol Reprod Biol, 2002, 104: 160−164.

②JANSEN F W, VREDEVOOGD C B, VAN ULZEN K, HERMANS J, TRIMBOS J B, TRIMBOS-KEMPER T C. Complications of hysteroscopy: a prospective, multicenter study. Obstet Gynecol, 2000, 96: 266−270.

③AGOSTINI A, CRAVELLO L, BRETELLE F, SHOJAI R, ROGER V, BLANC B. Risk of uterine perforation during hysteroscopic surgery. J Am Assoc Gynecol Laparosc, 2002, 9: 264−267.

④BRANDNER P, NEIS K J, EHMER C. The etiology, frequency, and prevention of gas embolism during CO_2 hysteroscopy. J Am Assoc Gynecol Laparosc, 1999, 6: 421−428.

⑤VILOS G A, HUTSON J R, SINGH I S, GIANNAKOPOULOS F, RAFEA B A, VILOS A G. Venous gas embolism during hysteroscopic endometrial ablation: report of 5 cases and review of the literature [published online May 14, 2019]. J Minim Invasive Gynecol. DOI: 10. 1016/j. jmig. 2019. 05. 003.

⑥ AGOSTINI A, CRAVELLO L, DESBRIERE R, MAISONNEUVE A S, ROGER V, BLANC B. Hemorrhage risk during operative hysteroscopy. Acta Obstet Gynecol Scand, 2002, 81: 878−881.

⑦AGOSTINI A, BRETELLE F, RONDA I, ROGER V, CRAVELLO L, BLANC B. Risk of vasovagal syndrome during outpatient hysteroscopy. J Am Assoc Gynecol Laparosc, 2004, 11: 245−247.

entry, which may increase the risk of uterine perforation. In a systematic review, the use of preoperative misoprostol reduced rates of false passage formation but did not reduce rates of uterine perforation during operative hysteroscopy[7]. Major bleeding, suspicion of visceral injury, or perforation by an electrosurgical electrode may warrant immediate surgical intervention.

Infection

Antibiotic prophylaxis is not recommended for routine hysteroscopic procedures. Hysteroscopy is contraindicated during an active pelvic infection[50] and in women with prodromal or active herpes infection. Infectious complications related to hysteroscopic procedures are uncommon with rates of postprocedure infection (eg, endometritis or endomyometritis, urinary tract infections) ranging from 0.01% to 1.42%[48, 51]. In a prospective observational study of 1,952 operative hysteroscopies, the risk of endometritis was found to be higher after adhesiolysis compared with leiomyoma (Relative Risk [RR], 5.89; CI, 1.68−20.69, $P=$ 0.0066) or polyp resection (RR, 6.36; CI, 1.3−31.24, $P=$0.0154)[52]. In randomized trials, the administration of antibiotic prophylaxis has not been shown to reduce postoperative infection after diagnostic hysteroscopy[53−55] or operative hysteroscopy[55].

Electrosurgical Injury

Serious injury by electrosurgical electrodes can occur during operative hysteroscopic procedures, typically in the setting of uterine perforation. Exploratory surgery may be indicated if clinically significant bleeding arises or if there is suspicion of thermal damage to visceral structures. Lower genital tract structures (eg, vagina or perineum) also may be at risk for thermal injury. Potential risk factors include cervical overdilation, instrument insulation defect, or electrode activation when the external sheath is not sufficiently advanced in the cervical canal[56].

Fluid Overload

See Box 2 for guidelines for fluid monitoring. Excessive absorption of distending fluid can result in severe complications, including pulmonary edema, neurologic complications, and death. Use of electrolyte-free, hypotonic distending media

Box 2. Guidelines for Fluid Monitoring and the Limits of Fluid Excess

1. Intravenous hydration of patients undergoing hysteroscopy should be closely monitored preoperatively and intraoperatively. Hysteroscopic fluid absorption should be closely monitored intraoperatively.

2. Lower fluid deficit thresholds should be considered for elderly patients, patients with comorbid conditions, patients with cardiovascular or renal compromise, and when procedures take place in an outpatient setting with limited acute care and laboratory services.

3. In healthy patients, the maximum fluid deficit is 1,000 mL for hypotonic solutions, 2,500 mL for isotonic solutions, and 500 mL for high-viscosity solutions. However, if fluid deficit reaches 750 mL of a hypotonic solution, 2,000 mL of an electrolyte solution, or 300 mL of a high-viscosity solution, consideration should be given to stopping further infusion and concluding the procedure. Ideally include the anesthesia personnel in this discussion, if applicable.

4. In an outpatient setting with limited acute care and laboratory services, consideration should be given to discontinuing procedures at a lower fluid deficit threshold.

5. An automated fluid monitoring system facilitates early recognition of excessive deficit in real-time totals.

6. An individual should be designated to measure intake and outflow frequently and report the deficit to the operative team.

7. If maximum fluid deficit occurs, especially with hypotonic solutions, evaluation of the patient's hemodynamic, neurologic, respiratory, and cardiovascular status is necessary along with assessment of signs and symptoms of fluid overload. Measurement of serum electrolytes and osmolality should be performed, administration of diuretics considered, and further diagnostic and therapeutic intervention begun as indicated. The use of intravenous furosemide may aid in diuresis, with clinical improvement occurring in 15−20 minutes. Further treatment of fluid overload or hyponatremia may require administration of corrective fluids, consultation with medical specialists, and transfer to a critical care setting.

Data from MUNRO M G, STORZ K, ABBOTT J A, FALCONE T, JACOBS V R, MUZII L, et al. AAGL practice report: practice guidelines for the management of hysteroscopic distending media: (replaces hysteroscopic fluid monitoring guidelines. J Am Assoc Gynecol Laparosc, 2000, 7: 167−168.) AAGL Advancing Minimally Invasive Gynecology Worldwide. J Minim Invasive Gynecol, 2013, 20: 137−148.

is associated with a greater risk of hypotonic hyponatremia and cerebral edema. Complications from fluid overload may be minimized with careful perioperative planning, use of a fluid management system, and evaluation of the intracavitary lesions to be removed. Fluid deficit is affected by size and number of the lesions removed, the depth of myometrial resection, the number of myometrial sinuses opened, and the intrauterine pressure. Preventive measures include limiting excess fluid absorption, recognizing and treating fluid overload promptly, and selecting a distending medium that minimizes risk. Vasopressin injection in the cervical stroma may reduce the volume of fluid intravasation[16]. The best way to limit excess fluid intravasation is to monitor the fluid deficit closely and frequently throughout the procedure. Management of fluid overload includes termination of procedure; assessment of hemodynamic, neurologic, respiratory and cardiovascular status; measurement of serum electrolytes and osmolality; and consideration of diuretic administration. Newer fluid management systems have made fluid monitoring more accurate; however, some of these systems may be expensive and not readily available in all settings.

Air and Gas Embolism

Air or gas embolism may result from the introduction of CO_2 as a hysteroscopic distending medium, room air during instrumentation of the cervix or uterus, gaseous byproducts created during monopolar or bipolar electrosurgery, or initial placement of patient in Trendelenburg position[57]. The chemical properties of gases affect the risk of embolism. The solubility of CO_2 in blood is higher than oxygen; therefore, the risk of an air embolism derived from room air (containing oxygen and nitrogen) is greater than the risk of a carbon dioxide gas embolism[58]. Severe complications of air or gas embolism include cardiac or pulmonary failure or death. The most common symptoms of air or gas embolism are described as dyspnea and chest pain, although in the anesthetized patient a decrease in end-tidal carbon dioxide pressure or alteration in hemodynamic status (hypotension, tachycardia) should raise clinical suspicion of an embolism event. A churning or splashing auscultatory sound (a "mill-wheel" murmur) is a classic physical examination finding, although it may not be detected in all cases. Although the reported incidences of emboli have been variable in the literature, the rate of clinically significant gas embolism is low[59, 60].

Risk reduction strategies for the prevention of air or gas embolism include purging air from hysteroscopic tubing and instruments; minimizing repetitive insertion of instruments through the cervix, which may introduce air into the uterus in a "piston-like" manner; removing intrauterine gas bubbles; and limiting intrauterine pressure. Acute management of air and gas embolism consists of both supportive care and active measures, including prompt termination of procedure, deflation of the uterine cavity, and the elimination of sources of fluid and gas. Durant's maneuver, described as placement of the patient in the left lateral decubitus and Trendelenburg position, can be performed to promote migration of air or gas toward the right ventricle to reduce obstruction at the right ventricular outflow tract[58].

Hemorrhage

For the management of hemorrhage, various intraoperative hemostasis measures can be employed, depending on the severity, nature, and location of bleeding; however, insufficient data exist regarding the effectiveness of these techniques. Examples include electrocautery applied to the source of bleeding, use of an intrauterine balloon (Foley catheter), uterine artery embolization, injection of vasopressin or epinephrine, tranexamic acid, and hysterectomy.

Vasovagal Reaction

Upon recognition of vasovagal signs (hypotension, bradycardia) or symptoms (nausea, vomiting, diaphoresis, pallor, or loss of consciousness), the procedure should be stopped and patient assessment and supportive care should be undertaken (vital signs including pulse and blood pressure and "ABCs" —airway, breathing, and circulation). The majority of vasovagal reactions resolve with supportive measures such as raising the patient's legs or placement in the Trendelenburg position. If symptoms or bradycardia persist, atropine may be administered as a single dosage of 0. 5 mg intravenously every 3 to 5 minutes, not to exceed a total of 3 mg[61].

References

[1] MUNRO M G, STORZ K, ABBOTT J A, FALCONE T, JACOBS V R, MUZII L, et al. AAGL practice report: practice guidelines for the management of hysteroscopic distending media: (replaces hysteroscopic fluid monitoring guidelines. JAm Assoc Gynecol Laparosc, 2000, 7: 167－168.). AAGL Advancing Minimally Invasive Gynecology Worldwide. J Minim Invasive Gynecol, 2013, 20: 137－148.

[2] KODAMA M, ONOUE M, OTSUKA H, YADA-HASHIMOTO N, SAEKI N, KODAMA T, et al. Efficacy of dienogest in thinning the endometrium before hysteroscopic surgery. J Minim Invasive Gynecol, 2013, 20: 790 －795.

[3] CICINELLI E, PINTO V, QUATTROMINI P, FUCCI M R, LEPERA A, MITOLA P C, et al. Endometrial preparation with estradiol plus dienogest (Qlaira) for office hysteroscopic polypectomy: randomized pilot study. J Minim Invasive Gynecol, 2012, 19: 356－359.

[4] LAGANA A S, VITALE S G, MUSCIA V, ROSSETTI P, BUSCEMA M, TRIOLO O, et al. Endometrial preparation with Dienogest before hysteroscopic surgery: a systematic review. Arch Gynecol Obstet, 2017, 295: 661 －667.

[5] KAMATH M S, KALAMPOKAS E E, KALAMPOKAS T E. Use of GnRH analogues pre-operatively for hysteroscopic resection of submucous fibroids: a systematic review and metaanalysis. Eur J Obstet Gynecol Reprod Biol, 2014, 177: 11－18.

[6] GKROZOU F, KOLIOPOULOS G, VREKOUSSIS T, VALASOULIS G, LAVASIDIS L, NAVROZOGLOU I, et al. A systematic review and meta-analysis of randomized studies comparing misoprostol versus placebo for cervical ripening prior to hysteroscopy. Eur J Obstet Gynecol Reprod Biol, 2011, 158:

17—23.

[7] AL-FOZAN H, FIRWANA B, AL-KADRI H, HASSAN S, TULAN-DI T. Preoperative ripening of the cervix before operative hysteroscopy. Cochrane Database of Systematic Reviews, 2015, Issue 4. Art. No. : CD005998. DOI: 10. 1002/14651858. CD005998. pub2.

[8] BASTU E, CELIK C, NEHIR A, DOGAN M, YUKSEL B, ERGUN B. Cervical priming before diagnostic operative hysteroscopy in infertile women: a randomized, double-blind, controlled comparison of 2 vaginal misoprostol doses. Int Surg, 2013, 98: 140—144.

[9] EL-MAZNY A, ABOU-SALEM N. A double-blind randomized controlled trial of vaginal misoprostol for cervical priming before outpatient hysteroscopy. Fertil Steril, 2011, 96: 962—965.

[10] ISSAT T, BETA J, NOWICKA M A, MACIEJEWSKI T, JAKIMI-UK A J. A randomized, single blind, placebo—controlled trial for the pain reduction during the outpatient hysteroscopy after ketoprofen or intravaginal misoprostol. J Minim Invasive Gynecol, 2014, 21: 921—927.

[11] CASADEI L, PICCOLO E, MANICUTI C, CARDINALE S, COLLAMARINI M, PICCIONE E. Role of vaginal estradiol pretreatment combined with vaginal misoprostol for cervical ripening before operative hysteroscopy in postmenopausal women. Obstet Gynecol Sci, 2016, 59: 220—226.

[12] OPPEGAARD K S, LIENG M, BERG A, ISTRE O, QVIGSTAD E, NESHEIM B I. A combination of misoprostol and estradiol for preoperative cervical ripening in postmenopausal women: a randomised controlled trial. BJOG, 2010, 117: 53—61.

[13] NADA A M, ELZAYAT A R, AWAD M H, METWALLY A A, TAHER A M, OGILA A I, et al. Cervical priming by vaginal or oral misoprostol before operative hysteroscopy: a double-blind, randomized controlled trial. J Minim Invasive Gynecol, 2016, 23: 1107—1112.

[14] LIN Y H, HWANG J L, SEOW K M, HUANG L W, CHEN H J, HSIEH B C. Laminaria tent vs misoprostol for cervical priming before hysteros-

copy: randomized study. J Minim Invasive Gynecol, 2009, 16: 708-712.

[15] PHILLIPS D R, NATHANSON H G, MILIM S J, HASELKORN J S, KHAPRA A, ROSS P L. The effect of dilute vasopressin solution on blood loss during operative hysteroscopy: a randomized controlled trial. Obstet Gynecol, 1996, 88: 761-766.

[16] PHILLIPS D R, NATHANSON H G, MILIM S J, HASELKORN J S. The effect of dilute vasopressin solution on the force needed for cervical dilatation: a randomized controlled trial. Obstet Gynecol, 1997, 89: 507-511.

[17] NEZHAT F, ADMON D, NEZHAT C H, DICORPO J E, NEZHAT C. Life-threatening hypotension after vasopressin injection during operative laparoscopy, followed by uneventful repeat laparoscopy. J Am Assoc Gynecol Laparosc, 1994, 2: 83-86.

[18] HOBO R, NETSU S, KOYASU Y, TSUTSUMI O. Bradycardia and cardiac arrest caused by intramyometrial injection of vasopressin during a laparoscopically assisted myomectomy. Obstet Gynecol, 2009, 113: 484-486.

[19] UGLIETTI A, BUGGIO L, FARELLA M, CHIAFFARINO F, DRIDI D, VERCELLINI P, et al. The risk of malignancy in uterine polyps: a systematic review and meta-analysis. Eur J Obstet Gynecol Reprod Biol, 2019, 237: 48-56.

[20] BETTOCCHI S, CECI O, VICINO M, MARELLO F, IMPEDOVO L, SELVAGGI L. Diagnostic inadequacy of dilatation and curettage. Fertil Steril, 2001, 75: 803-805.

[21] American Association of Gynecologic Laparoscopists. AAGL practice report: practice guidelines for the diagnosis and management of endometrial polyps. J Minim Invasive Gynecol, 2012, 19: 3-10.

[22] Alternatives to hysterectomy in the management of leiomyomas. ACOG Practice Bulletin No. 96. American College of Obstetricians and Gynecologists. Obstet Gynecol, 2008, 112: 387-400.

[23] WONG A S, CHEUNG C W, YEUNG S W, FAN H L, LEUNG T Y, SAHOTA D S. Transcervical intralesional vasopressin injection compared

with placebo in hysteroscopic myomectomy: a randomized controlled trial. Obstet Gynecol, 2014, 124: 897−903.

[24] TASKIN O, SADIK S, ONOGLU A, GOKDENIZ R, ERTURAN E, BURAK F, et al. Role of endometrial suppression on the frequency of intrauterine adhesions after resectoscopic surgery. J Am Assoc Gynecol Laparosc, 2000, 7: 351−354.

[25] YANG J H, CHEN M J, WU M Y, CHAO K H, HO H N, YANG Y S. Office hysteroscopic early lysis of intrauterine adhesion after transcervical resection of multiple apposing submucous myomas. Fertil Steril, 2008, 89: 1254 −1259.

[26] VAN DONGEN H, EMANUEL M H, SMEETS M J, TRIMBOS B, JANSEN F W. Follow-up after incomplete hysteroscopic removal of uterine fibroids. Acta Obstet Gynecol Scand, 2006, 85: 1463−1467.

[27] SMITH P P, MIDDLETON L J, CONNOR M, CLARK T J. Hysteroscopic morcellation compared with electrical resection of endometrial polyps: a randomized controlled trial. Obstet Gynecol, 2014, 123: 745−751.

[28] SHAZLY S A, LAUGHLIN-TOMMASO S K, BREITKOPF D M, HOPKINS M R, BURNETT T L, GREEN I C, et al. Hysteroscopic morcellation versus resection for the treatment of uterine cavitary lesions: a systematic review and meta-analysis. J Minim Invasive Gynecol, 2016, 23: 867−877.

[29] LI C, DAI Z, GONG Y, XIE B, WANG B. A systematic review and meta-analysis of randomized controlled trials comparing hysteroscopic morcellation with resectoscopy for patients with endometrial lesions. Int J Gynaecol Obstet, 2017, 136: 6−12.

[30] DEUTSCH A, SASAKI K J, CHOLKERI-SINGH A. Resectoscopic surgery for polyps and myomas: a review of the literature. J Minim Invasive Gynecol, 2017, 24: 1104−1110.

[31] KREMER C, DUFFY S, MORONEY M. Patient satisfaction with outpatient hysteroscopy versus day case hysteroscopy: randomised controlled trial. BMJ, 2000, 320: 279−282.

[32] MARSH F A, ROGERSON L J, DUFFY S R. A randomised controlled trial comparing outpatient versus daycase endometrial polypectomy. BJOG, 2006, 113: 896—901.

[33] DIWAKAR L, ROBERTS T E, COOPER N A, MIDDLETON L, JOWETT S, DANIELS J, et al. An economic evaluation of outpatient versus inpatient polyp treatment for abnormal uterine bleeding. BJOG, 2016, 123: 625—631.

[34] COOPER N A, CLARK T J, MIDDLETON L, DIWAKAR L, SMITH P, DENNY E, et al. Outpatient versus inpatient uterine polyp treatment for abnormal uterine bleeding: randomised controlled non-inferiority study. OPT Trial Collaborative Group. BMJ, 2015, 350: h1398.

[35] LUERTI M, VITAGLIANO A, DI SPIEZIO SARDO A, ANGIONI S, GARUTI G, DE ANGELIS C. Effectiveness of hysteroscopic techniques for endometrial polyp removal: The Italian Multicenter Trial. Italian School of Minimally Invasive Gynecological Surgery Hysteroscopists Group. J Minim Invasive Gynecol, 2019, 26: 1169—1176.

[36] Diagnosis of abnormal uterine bleeding in reproductiveaged women. Practice Bulletin No. 128. American College of Obstetricians and Gynecologists. Obstet Gynecol, 2012, 120: 197—206.

[37] COOPER N A, SMITH P, KHAN K S, CLARK T J. Vaginoscopic approach to outpatient hysteroscopy: a systematic review of the effect on pain [published erratum appears in BJOG, 2010, 117: 1440]. BJOG, 2010, 117: 532—539.

[38] SHARMA M, TAYLOR A, DI SPIEZIO SARDO A, BUCK L, MASTROGAMVRAKIS G, KOSMAS I, et al. Outpatient hysteroscopy: traditional versus the" no-touch" technique. BJOG, 2005, 112: 963—967.

[39] GARBIN O, KUTNAHORSKY R, GOLLNER J L, VAYSSIERE C. Vaginoscopic versus conventional approaches to outpatient diagnostic hysteroscopy: a two-centre randomized prospective study. Hum Reprod, 2006, 21: 2996—3000.

［40］SAGIV R, SADAN O, BOAZ M, DISHI M, SCHECHTER E, GO-LAN A. A new approach to office hysteroscopy compared with traditional hysteroscopy: a randomized controlled trial. Obstet Gynecol, 2006, 108: 387－392.

［41］Royal College of Obstetricians and Gynaecologists. Best practice in outpatient hysteroscopy. Green-top Guideline no. 59. London, UK: RCOG; 2011. Available at: https: //www. rcog. org. uk/globalassets/documents/guidelines/gtg59hysteroscopy. pdf. Retrieved November 8, 2019.

［42］JOHARY J, XUE M, XU B, XU D, AILI A. Use of hysteroscope for vaginoscopy or hysteroscopy in adolescents for the diagnosis and therapeutic management of gynecologic disorders: a systematic review. J Pediatr Adolesc Gynecol, 2015, 28: 29－37.

［43］AHMAD G, SALUJA S, O'FLYNN H, SORRENTINO A, LEACH D, WATSON A. Pain relief for outpatient hysteroscopy. Cochrane Database of Systematic Reviews, 2017, Issue 10. Art. No. : CD007710. DOI: 10. 1002/14651858. CD007710. pub3.

［44］KANESHIRO B, GRIMES D A, LOPEZ L M. Pain management for tubal sterilization by hysteroscopy. Cochrane Database of Systematic Reviews, 2012, Issue 8. Art. No. : CD009251. DOI: 10. 1002/14651858. CD009251. pub2.

［45］DE FREITAS FONSECA M, SESSA F V, RESENDE J A Jr, GUERRA C G, ANDRADE C M Jr, CRISPI C P. Identifying predictors of unacceptable pain at office hysteroscopy. J Minim Invasive Gynecol, 2014, 21: 586－591.

［46］American College of Obstetricians and Gynecologists. Report of the presidential task force on patient safety in the office setting. Washington, DC: American College of Obstetricians and Gynecologists; 2010.

［47］JANSEN F W, VREDEVOOGD C B, VAN ULZEN K, HERMANS J, TRIMBOS J B, TRIMBOS-KEMPER T C. Complications of hysteroscopy: a prospective, multicenter study. Obstet Gynecol, 2000, 96: 266－270.

［48］AYDENIZ B, GRUBER I V, SCHAUF B, KUREK R, MEYER A, WALLWIENER D. A multicenter survey of complications associated with 21,676 operative hysteroscopies. Eur J Obstet Gynecol Reprod Biol, 2002, 104: 160－164.

[49] AGOSTINI A, CRAVELLO L, BRETELLE F, SHOJAI R, ROGER V, BLANC B. Risk of uterine perforation during hysteroscopic surgery. J Am Assoc Gynecol Laparosc, 2002, 9: 264—267.

[50] Prevention of infection after gynecologic procedures. ACOG Practice Bulletin No. 195. American College of Obstetricians and Gynecologists. Obstet Gynecol, 2018, 131: e172—189.

[51] AGOSTINI A, CRAVELLO L, DESBRIERE R, MAISONNEUVE A S, ROGER V, BLANC B. Hemorrhage risk during operative hysteroscopy. Acta Obstet Gynecol Scand, 2002, 81: 878—881.

[52] AGOSTINI A, CRAVELLO L, SHOJAI R, RONDA I, ROGER V, BLANC B. Postoperative infection and surgical hysteroscopy. Fertil Steril, 2002, 77: 766—768.

[53] KASIUS J C, BROEKMANS F J, FAUSER B C, DEVROEY P, FATEMI H M. Antibiotic prophylaxis for hysteroscopy evaluation of the uterine cavity. Fertil Steril, 2011, 95: 792—794.

[54] GREGORIOU O, BAKAS P, GRIGORIADIS C, CREATSA M, SO-FOUDIS C, CREATSAS G. Antibiotic prophylaxis in diagnostic hysteroscopy: is it necessary or not? Eur J Obstet Gynecol Reprod Biol, 2012, 163: 190—192.

[55] NAPPI L, DI SPIEZIO SARDO A, SPINELLI M, GUIDA M, MEN-CAGLIA L, GRECO P, et al. A multicenter, doubleblind, randomized, placebo-controlled study to assess whether antibiotic administration should be recommended during office operative hysteroscopy. Reprod Sci, 2013, 20: 755—761.

[56] MUNRO M G. Mechanisms of thermal injury to the lower genital tract with radiofrequency resectoscopic surgery [published erratum appears in J Minim Invasive Gynecol, 2007, 14: 268]. J Minim Invasive Gynecol, 2006, 13: 36—42.

[57] BROOKS P G. Venous air embolism during operative hysteroscopy. J Am Assoc Gynecol Laparosc, 1997, 4: 399—402.

[58] GROENMAN F A, PETERS L W, RADEMAKER B M, BAKKUM E A. Embolism of air and gas in hysteroscopic procedures: pathophysiology and

implication for daily practice. J Minim Invasive Gynecol, 2008, 15: 241-247.

[59] BRANDNER P, NEIS K J, EHMER C. The etiology, frequency, and prevention of gas embolism during CO_2 hysteroscopy. J Am Assoc Gynecol Laparosc, 1999, 6: 421-428.

[60] DYRBYE B A, OVERDIJK L E, VAN KESTEREN P J, DE HAAN P, RIEZEBOS R K, BAKKUM E A, et al. Gas embolism during hysteroscopic surgery using bipolar or monopolar diathermia: a randomized controlled trial. Am J Obstet Gynecol, 2012, 207: 271, e1-e6.

[61] American Heart Association. Web-based integrated guidelines for cardiopulmonary resuscitation and emergency cardiovascular care-part 7: adult advanced cardiovascular life support. Dallas, TX: AHA; 2018. Available at: https://eccguidelines. heart. org/circulation/cpr-ecc-guidelines/part-7-adult-advanced-cardiovascular-life-support. Retrieved November 12, 2019.

Published online on February 20, 2020.

American College of Obstetricians and Gynecologists

409 12th Street SW, Washington, DC 20024-2188

The use of hysteroscopy for the diagnosis and treatment of intrauterine pathology. ACOG Committee Opinion No. 800. American College of Obstetricians and Gynecologists. Obstet Gynecol, 2020, 135: e138-48.

This information is designed as an educational resource to aid clinicians in providing obstetric and gynecologic care, and use of this information is voluntary. This information should not be considered as inclusive of all proper treatments or methods of care or as a statement of the standard of care. It is not intended to substitute for the independent professional judgment of the treating clinician. Variations in practice may be warranted when, in the reasonable judgment of the treating clinician, such course of action is indicated by the condition of the patient, limitations of available resources, or advances in knowledge or technology. The American College of Obstetricians and Gynecologists reviews its publications regularly; however, its publications may not reflect the most recent evidence. Any updates to this document can be found on acog. org or by calling the ACOG Resource Center.

While ACOG makes every effort to present accurate and reliable information, this publication is provided "as is" without any warranty of accuracy, reliability, or otherwise, either express or implied. ACOG does not guarantee, warrant, or endorse the products or services of any firm, organization, or person. Neither ACOG nor its officers, directors, members, employees, or agents will be liable for any loss, damage, or claim with respect to any liabilities, including direct, special, indirect, or consequential damages, incurred in connection with this publication or reliance on the information presented.

All ACOG committee members and authors have submitted a conflict of interest disclosure statement related to this published product. Any potential conflicts have been considered and managed in accordance with ACOG's Conflict of Interest Disclosure Policy. The ACOG policies can be found on acog. org. For products jointly developed with other organizations, conflict of interest disclosures by representatives of the other organizations are addressed by those organizations. The American College of Obstetricians and Gynecologists has neither solicited nor accepted any commercial involvement in the development of the content of this published product.

附录 B　欧洲妇科内镜学会（ESGE）
与 AAGL 联合发布子宫腔粘连临床指南

在发表前版的子宫腔粘连（IUA）的临床指南后，又有很多新的进展[1]。很多的临床结果为回顾性的研究。随机对照试验（RCT）论证了固体和半固态的屏障在预防一级和二级粘连中的应用，尽管没有非常严格地探讨不同的手术技术。最近的研究证明了不同时段的宫腔镜检查后，应用骨髓间充质干细胞技术均提高了妊娠结局。尽管在应用临床治疗之前，需要通过提供新的高质量数据来证明其有效性，这个结论同时可以提供新的研究方法。

一、背景

自 19 世纪末期到 20 世纪中期，子宫腔粘连作为继发性月经减少症状出现的原因已被证实[2]。Asherman 进一步描述了妊娠后发生的类似情况[3,4]，人们命名为"阿谢曼（Asherman）综合征"，它与 IUA 经常互换使用，尽管综合征需要有一系列相关的症状和体征（例如疼痛、月经紊乱、生育能力低下等）来支持诊断，这些是与子宫腔粘连相关的症状[3,4]。若无症状出现，最好是归为无症状性 IUA，并探讨它的临床意义。在这些指南中我们应用 IUA 这个术语，特异性地指出它是否与临床症状相关。

二、证据的鉴定和评估

AAGL 的临床指南通过研究电子数据库而制定，包括 Medline、PubMed、CINAHL、实证医学资料库（包括系统评价的研究数据库）、最新的期刊目录和 EMBASE，以及自 2016 年 4 月以前所有与 IUA 相关的文献。查 MeSH（MED-LARS）术语，包括：副标题和关键字中含有 Asherman 综合征；子宫腔粘连；子宫纵隔和子宫粘连；宫腔镜下粘连松解术；宫腔镜检查和粘连以及宫腔内手术后的产科结局。

此项研究不只限定于英文文献；委员会成员中擅长非英语的人员翻译和解释了相关的文献。所有有电子数据存储的文献均包括在研究的范围内，以及相关的电子产品（如在电子数据开始使用之前出版的材料）被交叉引用手工搜索数目，包括在文献中审查。有时为了进一步明确一些数据，我们直接联系作者进行核对。所有的研究都应用严格的方法学进行评估，并且根据美国联邦预防医学工作组分类系统进行分级。IUA 是根据之前的美国联邦预防医学工作组分类系统进行临床指南概述[1]。在可能的情况下，建议是基于现有的最佳证据，若没有这样的证据，就基于专家小组的一致同意决定。

三、诊断

Asherman 综合征的女性体检经常并未发现异常[5,6]。盲目的经宫颈探查在宫颈内口或附近可能会遇到阻力[6]；而宫腔内位置较高或者两侧壁的粘连不能用这种方法来判断。宫腔镜为检查 IUA 的金标准[7]。与放射性检查对照，在探查宫腔时，宫腔镜检查更准确地发现粘连的位置、程度和它的形态学特征以及子宫内膜质量。宫腔镜可以实时地察看宫腔，能够准确地描述粘连的位置程度并同时处理 IUA[8]。

输卵管造影（HSG）应用对照的染料，其敏感性为 $75\%\sim81\%$，特异性为 80%，与宫腔镜检查诊断 IUA 对照，阳性预测值为 50%[9,10]，有较高的假阳性预测值（达 39%）[11]，因此限制了这种方法的应用。它也不能检查子宫内膜的纤维化情况[4]或者 IUA 的程度[12]，这也就是筛查监测中限制使用此方法的原因。

灌注盐水或胶溶液的超声检查（Sonohysterography，SHG）效果与 HST 差不多。SHG 和 HSG 同样有效，两种检查方法都有 75% 敏感度，与宫腔镜相比，SHG 阳性率约为 43%，HSG 阳性率约为 50%[10,13]。与宫腔镜相比，阴道 2D 超声敏感性和特异性分别是 52% 和 11%[13]。3D 超声对 IUAs 的诊断性更高，与 3D SHG 相比它的敏感性和特异性分别为 87% 和 45%（尽管此项研究未与宫腔镜检查对照）[14]。和标准的宫腔镜相比，3D SHG 特异性为 87%，而敏感性稍低一点，为 70%[15]。

最近较新的技术包括多普勒超声发现，高的血流阻抗与差的产科结局相关联[16]，以及彩色能量血管造影成像的 3D 超声技术可能在 Asherman 综合征的形成和预后方面发挥作用[17]。与其他价格低廉的检查方法相比，磁共振成像检查（MRI）在初始评估 IUA 时显示很少的优势[18-20]，与普通 MRI 相比，最近应用的增强图像在 IUA 诊断上更加有前景[21,22]。没有任何一项技术可以完全的用来评估或被推荐作为常规诊断方法来推广，除非有更进一步的研究来证明[23]。

子宫腔粘连的诊断指南

1. 宫腔镜为诊断子宫腔粘连的金标准，应该尽可能地通过此技术来明确诊断（B级）。

2. 如果无法行宫腔镜检查，HSG 和 SGH 也可以用来诊断（B级）。

3. 除了临床研究，MRI 不应该用来诊断（C级）。

四、分类

分类对于评估疾病严重程度和预后有关[8]。IUA 有很多分类系统，每一种都包括宫腔镜下粘连的特征[24]。到目前为止，还没有任何的数据提供分析这些分类系统之间的对比。附表 B-1 给出了分类系统和它们的主要特征。

子宫腔粘连的分类指南

1. 子宫腔粘连应该根据与预后相关的严重程度来分类（B级）。

2. 两个研究之间的对比很难用多种分类系统来解释。这可能反映在不同的分类系统内在的缺陷方面。因此，最近不可能签署任何专门的系统（C级）。

附表 B-1　子宫腔粘连的分类

来源	分类方法概要
March 等[7]	根据宫腔镜评估子宫腔受累程度，将粘连分为轻度、中度或重度
Hamou 等[25]	根据宫腔镜评估，将粘连分为峡部、边缘、中心或重度
Valle 和 Sciarra[26]	根据宫腔镜评估和在 HSG 下闭塞的面积（部分或全部），将粘连分为轻度、中度或重度
欧洲宫腔镜学会[27]	根据宫腔镜和 HSG 结果和临床症状相结合，将粘连分为 I 到 IV 的几个亚型的复杂系统
美国生育学会[28]	根据宫腔镜或 HSG 看到的子宫内膜腔闭塞程度、粘连现象和患者月经情况，将粘连分为轻度、中度或重度的复杂评分系统
Donnez 和 Nisolle[29]	以位置、术后妊娠率为主要因素将粘连分为 6 个级别。用宫腔镜或 HSG 进行评估
Nasr 等[30]	将月经和产科史与子宫腔粘连结果并入宫腔镜评估来创建预后评分的复杂系统

五、一级预防

有 8 个关于 IUA 术后一级预防的 RCT 研究[31-38]。第一个 RCT 评估了宫腔镜整形术后口服雌激素的价值，结果提示，它对术后新的粘连形成没有太多意义[31]。术后女性每天口服 2 mg 戊酸雌二醇，连用 30 天后用宫腔镜二探，发现 42 人无粘连，而对照组中有 3 人（3/43，7％）发生子宫腔粘连。在随后 2 年的随访中，二者的妊娠率没有明显差异（雌二醇和对照组分别为 37％和 41％）。另一组 RCT 中有相似的报道，100 个宫腔镜修复术后的患者，给予以下几种处理：①没有任何处置；②单独应用雌激素；③雌激素＋放置宫内节育器；④单独放置宫内节育器[32]。术后评估，几种方法在新粘连形成和妊娠结局方面没有明显的差异。

其他六个 RCT 评估了术后应用半固体胶的作用[33-38]。由于其高敏感性和长时间作用于受损的子宫内膜表面，适用于预防 IUA[39]。研究中，随机分配控制组和对照组，控制组包括为聚乙烯氧化钠羧基甲基纤维素胶和透明质酸钠衍生物，或者二者互为对照。其中两项研究发现放置胶组明显降低了粘连的再形成（两个实验中两组的粘连形成情况分别为 3/55（5％）和 12/55（22％）[33]；7/67（10％）和 17/65（26％）[35]。两组观察中 $P<0.05$，但与妊娠情况无关。还有一组观察，在双盲分组后，术后 9 周随访行中，处理组和对照组中发现没有粘连的情况分别为 13/18（72％）和 15/22（68％）[38]。尽管无统计学意义，但是发现对照组的粘连情况要重于处理组。遗憾的是，没有文献报道随后的妊娠情况。

这些 RCT 中的第六个研究中，随访宫腔镜下去妊娠残留物后应用屏障作为初级预防的患者的情况，在术后平均 20 个月的随访中，术后 6～8 周行二探术，中重度粘连的女性处理组和对照组的差异没有统计学意义 [1 例（4％）给予了屏障处理，另 3 例（14％）是控制组患者；$P=0.3$]。随后的妊娠情况为屏障组 7 例（27％），而控制组为 3 例（14％）（$P=0.5$）[34]。第七个研究中，随访了 150 例因不全流产、过期流产和习惯性流产而行吸宫术的女性[36]。其中 50 人随机地给予了屏障性的防粘连处理，100 人作为控制组。在实验组，32 人（100％）在 8 个月内妊娠，而控制组中有 34 人（54％）妊娠。未妊娠的女性中，处理组中 1 例（1/10，10％）发生粘连，而控制组中有 7 例（7/14，50％）再次发生了粘连。处理组没有发生不良事件。

第八个 RCT 中，187 例不同类型的子宫腔粘连术后应用澡胺素透明质酸钠和透明质酸钠对比没有发现他们对于预防粘连有什么差异，尽管研究发现澡胺素透明质酸钠可以作为好的预防粘连的产品（$P=0.02$）[37]。

回顾性的研究发现手术的方式可能影响粘连形成，宫腔镜或者超声引导下手术强于盲目[40-42]的刮宫术[43]。然而，这些研究也指出对于尽早再次妊娠的情况，还缺乏进一步评估的方法学支持。宫腔镜手术的类型也可能影响预后和粘连的形成[44]。前瞻性的研究发现，子宫内膜息肉切除术后子宫内膜修复最快，而子宫腔纵隔术后修复最慢[45]。粘连发生率最低的是子宫内膜息肉切除术，最高的为多发性的子宫黏膜下肌瘤电切术。避免应用宫腔镜下电外科模式切除子宫肌瘤可能是预防宫腔镜粘连的最重要的方式，对此已有对肌瘤切除术后粘连形成部位的周围组织进行病理检测的报道[46-48]。最近大的回顾性的队列研究已经发表，指出在宫腔镜下切除子宫肌瘤手术中应用冷刀结合尽可能少的射频电能技术可以降低子宫腔粘连的发生率（4%）[47]。

子宫腔粘连的初级预防指南

1. 宫腔镜手术类型可以影响新粘连形成。仅限于子宫内膜表面的手术，例如息肉切除术，形成粘连的概率最低，而侵犯子宫内膜内层或者损伤病变对侧的组织，发生粘连的概率将增加（B 级）。

2. 手术的方式影响新粘连的形成。非妊娠状态下电外科手术和妊娠状态下盲目刮宫的风险是最高的操作（C 级）。

3. 术后应用屏障性防粘连材料短期内可以使损伤的子宫内膜明显降低粘连的再次形成，尚缺乏干预后妊娠情况的研究数据（A 级）。

六、治疗

IUA 并非致命性疾病，只有那些有体征或疼痛、不孕症、习惯性流产或者月经异常包括宫腔积血的患者需要治疗。手术是治疗 Asherman 综合征的金标准。然而，没有 RCT 对照手术和期待疗法的研究，也没有 RCT 对照不同的手术方法治疗 Asherman 综合征的情况的研究。任何干预都是为了恢复宫腔和宫颈管的体积和形状，以便保持宫腔与宫颈管和输卵管的联通。这样保障了正常月经和大量精子的穿过，利于受精和种植。

1. 期待治疗：目前这方面的观察数据有限，1982 年发表的数据表明，从诊断为 IUA 到月经恢复，78％的人在 7 年内恢复月经周期，有 45.5％的人妊娠[49]。

2. 宫颈探查：若宫腔未受累，仅有宫颈管狭窄，超声引导下探针探测宫颈管即可[50]。在宫腔镜指引下分离粘连出现之前，收集所有可利用的数据，有报道称盲探宫颈发生子宫穿孔的情况，这种操作目前也没有被大力推广。

3. 诊断性刮宫：宫腔镜普及之前，诊刮是处理此类问题的主要方式，报道 84％（1049/1250）的女性恢复了月经，流产率为 25％（142/559），足月产 55％（306/559），早产为 9％（50/559），妊娠合并胎盘植入的为 8％（42/559）[49]。此研究中，粘连程度不详，可能大多数为轻度。随着宫腔镜技术的普及，诊刮术应该废弃，精确诊断和分类不应该进一步损伤子宫内膜。

4. 宫腔镜：宫腔镜技术可以直视下分解粘连。对于轻度粘连，可以用镜子本身分解，钝性分离可以用镜子头端操作[51]。侧壁粘连越多，密度越大，分离越困难，发生子宫穿孔等并发症的可能性越大[4,52]。单极[26,53-56]、双极[57-59]和 Nd-YAG 激光[26,54,60]等电设备常用于粘连分解，具有可视引导、精确的切割和良好的止血效果等优势。它的缺点包括发生子宫穿孔后潜在的脏器损伤[8]；进一步的子宫内膜损伤更容易形成 IUA[61,62]；宫颈扩张需要合适的手术器械，增加了费用。这些技术之间没有对照的研究，所以不能说哪一种方法是更好。有间接的证据指出尽量少应用电设备分解粘连，因为可能会进一步加重子宫内膜的损伤[63]。手术可以采用剪刀[7,26]和针[64,65]机械分离粘连。手术可以在门诊或住院完成，结果没有差异[66]。

5. 其他宫腔镜技术：当典型的宫腔镜直视下不能完成重度致密粘连的手术时，切开子宫肌层对于扩大子宫腔大小是一个很有效的方法。用 collins 刀电极从宫底到宫颈划 6～8 个 4 mm 深的切口可以扩大子宫腔的容积。一项研究表明，71％的患者恢复了宫腔解剖，其中 3 个人妊娠（3/7，42.9％）[67]，另一个研究[53]有 51.6％的人恢复解剖结构，12 人随后妊娠（12/31 38.7％）。

6. 宫腔镜其他指导技术：透视指导下钝性分离重度粘连的患者是在全身麻醉后，给予图像增强剂控制并在宫腔镜指引下用 Tuohy 针进行分离[64]。它的费用很高，且患者需要暴露于电离辐射中，对技术的要求很高。它的优点是镜子很窄，降低了子宫穿孔和由此带来的脏器损伤，且不需要使用能量器械[65,68]。另一个相似的技术是在局部麻醉下用一个流动的设备完成轻度子宫腔粘连的手术治疗[69]。

腹部超声可以作为检测宫腔镜手术的一个方法[4,62,67,70,71]。超声检测可以在无创的条件下监测宫腔镜手术；即便如此，仍有 5% 的病例发生了子宫穿孔[58,67,72]。腹腔镜监测对于重度子宫腔粘连的患者也是另一种方法，它可以同时观察盆腔脏器的情况[58,67,72]。

还有人报道对于宫腔闭塞性粘连处置是放置宫颈扩张器，从宫颈管一直到 2 个开口处，产生 2 个侧壁的标志和一个中央的纤维纵隔，然后在腹腔镜监护下宫腔镜下将其分开。6 个病例被报道 2 个人发生了子宫穿孔，另一例发生了大出血[72]。虽然提高了妊娠情况，但是样本数量极少，腹腔镜监护等增加了费用及增加了潜在的并发症等发生，此项技术不予推广。

7. 非宫腔镜的方法治疗子宫腔粘连：传统地处理重度子宫腔粘连，通常开腹行子宫切开术用手指或搔刮钝性分离粘连[6,50,58,62]。有一个 31 例和几个个案报道用这种方法处理，妊娠率为 52%（16/31），11 例活产（38%），包括 8 例足月产（26%）。16 例妊娠病例中，5 例（31%）合并胎盘植入[49]。目前临床中，很少应用此方法，只有没有其他可替代的方法时才考虑此项技术[73]。

8. 宫腔粘连的手术治疗指南：

（1）对有症状的子宫腔粘连，手术方式包括宫腔镜可视下直接分离和用工具分离两种（B 级）。

（2）没有证据支持使用宫颈盲探（C 级）。

（3）没有证据支持宫腔盲扩和盲刮（C 级）。

（4）对于不想进行任何干预的有生育要求的女性，期待疗法仍可以妊娠，但是可能间期会比较长（C 级）。

（5）辅助完成子宫腔粘连分离的技术包括超声，X 线透视（荧光镜检查）和腹腔镜检查。没有研究表明这些辅助技术可以防止子宫穿孔或者提高手术结果，最终的疗效还要根据临床技能和它的有效性。然而，若采取这种方式，必须选择恰当的病例，这样才能最大限度地减少子宫穿孔的发生（B 级）。

（6）当发现广泛和致密粘连的情况，应该由有经验的宫腔镜专家来处理（C 级）。

七、二级预防

已经行子宫腔粘连分解术后的患者，再次发生粘连的概率为 30%～66%。大量的随机试验评估术后放置各种不同类型的固体或半固体屏障预防粘连复发[26,53,74~76]。传统的防粘连使用固体的设备分隔子宫壁，例如粘连分解术后放置 IUD，新鲜羊膜或者扩张，最典型的是宫腔内放置尖端带球囊的尿管。术后放置胶体，如透明质酸钠和聚乙烯羧甲基纤维素也受到更严格的调查，总共 5 相关目前评估结果为二级预防策略。

1. 固体屏障：子宫腔粘连分离术后放置 IUD 分隔子宫内膜层已经应用于临床多年[7,49,77]。含铜和 T 形 IUD 因为导致炎性反应特性[78]和接触面小[79]不推荐临床应用。可选择放置惰性环形 IUD（例如 Lippes 环）[4]，尽管在一些地区已经不再应用。在一个前瞻性对照研究中，71 位女性在行子宫腔粘连分解术后放置 Lippes 环并给予雌孕激素治疗 2 个月后二探[77]。第一组患者术后 1 周行宫腔镜检查，2 个月后取出 IUD 后再次评估；第二组于术后 1 周再探。两组在妊娠率和活产率方面无差异并且未与没放 IUD 的女性进行比较。一个随机对照研究对比了 80 例放置 IUD 和 82 例放置球囊的患者术后情况，术后放置 1 周后取出[80]。术后 1~2 个月行宫腔镜检查对粘连情况进行评分，结果发现两组无明显差异（放置球囊组为 30%，IUD 组为 35%）。此研究未报道妊娠结果或者没有术后干预的对照。有一个小型非随机对照观察，术后放置 IUD 和给予激素治疗与术后单独给予激素治疗对照，发现两种处理对于术后粘连的再次形成没有明显差异[81]。术后直接放置 IUD 后致感染的风险估计为 8%[82]，也有报道因放置 IUD 而致子宫穿孔的病例[82]。

子宫腔粘连分解术后放置尿管 3~10 天的效果类似于宫腔内放置屏障保护[7,50,56,69,83,84]。非随机对照试验对比了 59 例术后应用儿童 Foley 尿管 10 天和 51 例放置 IUD 3 个月的女性[82]，研究发现，放置尿管组很少发生感染，应用 HSG 评估发现放置 IUD 组粘连复发率低[82]。尽管两组闭经率分别为 19%（尿管组）和 38%（IUD 组），两组的妊娠率相对低，尿管组为 34%（20/59），IUD 组为 28%（14/51）。一项对 25 名中重度粘连的女性观察中，应用新鲜羊膜放于尿管表面，防止了 52% 的患者 IUA 复发，尽管没有报道随后的妊娠和并发症情况[83]。

一项三臂实验评估新鲜羊膜，干羊膜和宫腔内放置球囊的随机对照试验[85]。45 名女性平均分配到三个组中（每组 15 例患者）。每组患者诊断性宫腔镜手术后 2~4 个月随访。羊膜组的再次粘连明显好于球囊组（$P<0.003$），新鲜羊膜组

由于干羊膜组（$P<0.05$）。10 例（23％）妊娠，其中 6 例（60％）流产。

一个 60 个样本的 RCT 实验（30 名女性接受宫腔内放置支架类物质，30 人作为对照组）评估了有关感染的情况[86]。宫腔镜术后 30 天，应用细菌培植法评估感染情况。结果发现，两者之间没有明显差异（术前术后的细菌培养率未放支架组分别为 13％和 33％，放支架组分别为 10％和 30％）。也就是是否感染与宫腔内放置支架没有明显的关系。

2. 半固体屏障：很多研究报道宫腔镜粘连分解术后，应用半固体胶可以降低粘连再次形成[35,36,87]。自动十字铰链透明质酸钠因对受损的内膜的高度敏感性和延长受损表面组织保护的时间，更适合预防子宫腔粘连[39]。84 例样本的 RCT 观察术后放胶与不放胶的对照研究。术后超声检查证实放胶组术后 72 小时，子宫壁保持分离。3 个月后二探，宫腔粘连明显低于对照组 ［6/43（14％）和 13/41（32％）；（$P<0.05$）[87]］。妊娠情况未予报道。

一项回顾性的研究对照组与球囊，IUD，透明质酸钠对比，发现球囊在降低粘连方面较其他方法效果好（$P<0.001$）。IUD 组比胶的效果好（$P<0.001$），也好于对照组（$P<0.001$），而宫腔内放置胶和对照组比较没有差异[88]。

来源于随机对照的动物实验数据发现应用透明质酸钠可以提供术后妊娠率[89]，也就是术后使用胶屏障处理可以降低再粘连的形成，并提高妊娠率。

3. 激素治疗：术后应用雌激素（每天给予结合雌激素 2.5 mg，加或不加孕激素 2～3 个周期）[24,64,65,73] 已有报道，无不同剂量，处理或者结合激素的研究。一个非随机对照研究报告单独的应用激素的效果等同于激素连同 IUD 处理[81]。

4. 增加子宫内膜血流的技术：很多研究应用药物，如阿司匹林，硝酸甘油[90-93]和西地那非柠檬酸盐增加子宫内膜血管的灌流[94]。然而，此研究的人群数目有限，而且所有的这些处理都是临床未予认证的药物，这些药物不能被严格的研究项目以外的范围应用。

5. 抗生素应用：之前没有证据支持术后应用抗生素。美国妇产科协会不推荐宫腔镜术后应用抗生素[95]。然而，理论上有再次感染的风险，IUA 也被认为是感染后粘连形成的主要原因。这就导致了一些外科医生在宫腔粘连松解术前或术中给予抗生素，一些人在术后继续给予抗生素治疗。然而，目前没有证据支持或否定抗生素的治疗效果。

6. 干细胞治疗宫腔粘连技术：曾经有一段时间，人们假定应用人干细胞重建受损和 IUA 形成的子宫内膜[96]，有关这方面的动物模型的研究显示了此领域医学治疗方面有大量的前景可言[97-99]。从人类的第一个前瞻性研究，16 个患者用宫腔镜确认为 IUA，静脉内注射 BMDSC[100]。临床上，报道宫腔镜后注射 BMDSC 后 6 个月，月经功能恢复正常，有 3 个自然妊娠，7 个 IVF 成功。这些原始数据来自人类的事件，这样的治疗方法是对 Asherman 的第一次辅助治疗成功地调整了月经和妊娠结局。当前，首要的任务是妥善地建立 BMDSC 在除了手术或单独手术治疗之前的角色的随机对照试验。

7. 二级预防宫腔粘连的指南：

（1）IUD，支架或尿管降低了术后粘连的形成。没有更多的证据表明这些对于后期的妊娠结果的影响（A 级）。

（2）固体屏障感染的概率最小（A 级）。

（3）没有证据支持或反驳术前、术中、术后使用抗生素（C 级）。

（4）术后应该放置表面积大的 IUD，例如 Lippes 环。子宫腔粘连术后不应该放置含孕激素和含铜的 IUD（C 级）。

（5）半固体屏障例如透明质酸钠和自动交联的透明质酸钠可以降低再次粘连的形成。目前，它们对于治疗后妊娠率情况还不知道（A 级）。

（6）宫腔镜指导下宫腔粘连分解术后，用雌激素治疗，用或不用孕激素，可减低粘连的复发（B 级）。

（7）辅助性用药提高子宫内膜血管血流的作用仍无法知晓。因此它们不应该在严格的研究设计之外应用（C 级）。

（8）干细胞治疗可能最终提供一个有效的治疗 Asherman 综合征的辅助方法；然而，对此的研究非常有限，不应该在严格的试验设计之外应用（C 级）。

8. 术后评估：1/3 轻中度子宫腔粘连的女性复发[26,74,75]，而重度粘连有 2/3 复发[53,76]。因此，不管是否进行外科干预，宫腔的再评估是有价值的，通常在术后 2~3 个月经周期后进行评估[53]。动态评估包括门诊宫腔镜检查和 HSG，高于轻度粘连可能需要麻醉下分离。随机[75]的前瞻性和回顾性研究[99,100]均建议宫腔镜术后几周而不是几个月进行评估。

9. 子宫腔粘连治疗术后评估指南：推荐进行子宫腔粘连治疗后的术后随访，最好是用宫腔镜进行（B 级）。

八、结果

判断子宫腔粘连症状治疗结果包括粘连评分，月经周期，生育率和临床表现。目前已发表的大型数据主要是回顾性的。据报道，最好的生育结果是一位外科医生在 674/807 名（84％）妇女中报告了活产，虽然在这份报告中手术治疗的总数是未知的[101]。回顾性分析了 683 例中重度粘连患者，术后使用包括宫内节育器、球囊、雌激素和透明质酸在内的一种或一种联合佐剂，妊娠率为 314/475（66％），其中 201/314（61％）活产[102]。荷兰的一个全国性转诊中心报告了 638 名连续治疗的妇女在 10 年内的月经结果[68]。以正常月经作为判断成功的概率为 95％。然而，其中 27％的女性在最多 3 次外科操作后有子宫腔粘连的复发，而那些在基线时粘连更严重的人更有可能需要随后的粘连松解术。子宫腔粘连发展的病因似乎也会影响结果。有子宫腔粘连的妇女联合子宫动脉栓塞[103]或子宫压迫缝线者似乎比具有继发于子宫内手术创伤的粘连更有利的结果[104,105]。对使用凝胶屏障者进行 meta 分析指出生育结果一般质量差[106]。一个主要问题是，RCT检查这种干预主要报告了减少粘连改变，而不是随后的妊娠。这些汇总的数据在这个时候并不意味着任何生育结果的好处，而对于今后的研究报告这些数据至关重要。

九、对未来研究的建议

根据以前的指南，有越来越多的随机对照试验，尤其是一级和二级预防的评价方法。具体的手术技术仍然未经 RCT 测试，但是已经认识到了合并手术改变、方案制订、遵循和补充问题的子宫腔粘连治疗的这一方面将很难调查的问题。具体的未来研究途径可能包括：

1. 可能预示结果的诊断方法，包括造影剂、3D 重建、多普勒或血流研究和 MRI 技术在内的超声检查可以为考虑治疗的妇女提供咨询时为治疗预后和价值提供新的途径。

2. 从一级和二级预防技术的随机对照试验中论证的生育结果，目前子宫腔粘连产生的最重要也是最常见的影响是不孕。

3. 基于初步研究，进一步研究骨髓间充质干细胞治疗作为手术的替代手段。

我们认为，通用分类系统将有利于未来的研究，尽管考虑到当前任何单一分类系统的局限性，这在可预见的未来不可能发生。

冯力民

【参考文献】

[1] MUNRO M G, ABBOTT J A, BRADLEY L D, et al. AAGL practice report: prac-tice guidelines for management of intrauterine synechiae. J Minim Invasive Gynecol, 2010, 17: 1-7.

[2] FRITSCH H. Ein fall von voelligem schwund der gebarmutterhoehle nach auskratzung. Zentralbl Gynakol, 1894, 18: 1337-1339.

[3] ASHERMAN J G. Amenorrhoea traumatica (atretica). J Obstet Gynaecol Br Emp, 1948, 55: 23-30.

[4] YU D, WONG Y M, CHEONG Y, et al. Asherman syndrome: one century later. Fertil Steril, 2008, 89: 759-779.

[5] JONES W E. Traumatic intrauterine adhesions: a report of 8 cases with emphasis on therapy. Am J Obstet Gynecol, 1964, 89: 304-313.

[6] NETTER A P, MUSSET R, LAMBERT A, et al. Traumatic uterine synechiae: a common cause of menstrual insufficiency, sterility, and abortion. Am J Obstet Gynecol, 1956, 71: 368-375.

[7] MARCH C M, ISRAEL R, MARCH A D. Hysteroscopic management of intra-uterine adhesions. Am J Obstet Gynecol, 1978, 130: 653-657.

[8] MAGOS A. Hysteroscopic treatment of Asherman's syndrome. Reprod Biomed Online, 2002, 4 (suppl 3): 46-51.

[9] ROMA DALFO A, UBEDA B, UBEDA A, et al. Diagnostic value of hysterosal-pingography in the detection of intrauterine abnormalities: a comparison with hysteroscopy. AJR Am J Roentgenol, 2004, 183: 1405-1409.

[10] SOARES S R, BARBOSA DOS REIS M M, CAMARGOS A F. Diagnostic accuracy of sonohysterography, transvaginal sonography, and hysterosalpingography in patients with uterine cavity diseases. Fertil Steril, 2000, 73: 406-411.

[11] RAZIEL A, ARIELI S, BUKOVSKY I, et al. Investigation of the u-

terine cavity in recurrent aborters. Fertil Steril, 1994, 62: 1080−1082.

[12] FAYEZ J A, MUTIE G, SCHNEIDER P J. The diagnostic value of hysterosal-pingography and hysteroscopy in infertility investigation. Am J Obstet Gynecol, 1987, 156: 558−560.

[13] SALLE B, GAUCHERAND P, DE SAINT HILAIRE P, et al. Transvaginal sonohysterographic evaluation of intrauterine adhesions. J Clin Ultrasound, 1999, 27: 131−134.

[14] SYLVESTRE C, CHILD T J, TULANDI T, et al. A prospective study to eval-uate the efficacy of two-and three-dimensional sonohysterography in women with intrauterine lesions. Fertil Steril, 2003, 79: 1222−1225.

[15] LAGANÀ A S, CIANCIMINO L, MANCUSO A, et al. 3D sonohysterography vs hysteroscopy: a cross-sectional study for the evaluation of endo-uterine diseases. Arch Gynecol Obstet, 2014, 290: 1173−1178.

[16] MALHOTRA N, BAHADUR A, KALAIVANI M, et al. Changes in endometrial receptivity in women with Asherman's syndrome undergoing hysteroscopic adhesiolysis. Arch Gynecol Obstet, 2012, 286: 525−530.

[17] YAN L, WANG A, BAI R, et al. Application of SonoVue combined with three-dimensional color power angiography in the diagnosis and prognosis e-valuation of intrauterine adhesion. Eur J Obstet Gynecol Reprod Biol, 2016, 198: 68−72.

[18] BACELAR A C, WILCOCK D, POWELL M, et al. The value of MRI in the assessment of traumatic intra-uterine adhesions (Asherman's syndrome). Clin Radiol, 1995, 50: 80−83.

[19] DYKES T A, ISLER R J, MCLEAN A C. MR imaging of Asherman syndrome: total endometrial obliteration. J Comput Assist Tomogr, 1991, 15: 858−860.

[20] LETTERIE G S, HAGGERTY M F. Magnetic resonance imaging of intrauterine synechiae. Gynecol Obstet Invest, 1994, 37: 66−68.

[21] HUANG S M, GAO J F, SHI L J, et al. A preliminary study of the relationship between the uterine junction zone and outcome of intrauterine adhe-

sions. Med J China PLA, 2016, 41: 301−306.

[22] WOLFMAN D J, ASCHER S M. Magnetic resonance imaging of benign uterine pathology. Top Magn Reson Imaging, 2006, 17: 399−407.

[23] TAKEUCHI M, MATSUZAKI K, NISHITANI H. Diffusion-weighted magnetic resonance imaging of endometrial cancer: differentiation from benign endometrial lesions and preoperative assessment of myometrial invasion. Acta Radiol, 2009, 50: 947−953.

[24] KODAMAN P H, ARICI A. Intra-uterine adhesions and fertility outcome: how to optimize success? Curr Opin Obstet Gynecol, 2007, 19: 207−214.

[25] HAMOU J, SALAT-BAROUX J, SIEGLER A M. Diagnosis and treatment of intrauterine adhesions by microhysteroscopy. Fertil Steril, 1983, 39: 321−326.

[26] VALLE R F, SCIARRA J J. Intrauterine adhesions: hysteroscopic diagnosis, classification, treatment, and reproductive outcome. Am J Obstet Gynecol, 1988, 158: 1459−1470.

[27] WAMSTEKER K, DE BLOK S J. Diagnostic hysteroscopy: technique and documentation//SUTTON C, DIAMON M, editors. Endoscopic Surgery for Gynecologists. New York: Lippincott Williams & Wilkins Publishers, 1995: 263−276.

[28] The American Fertility Society. Classifications of adnexal adhesions, distal tubal occlusion, tubal occlusion secondary to tubal ligation, tubal pregnancies, mullerian anomalies and intrauterine adhesions. Fertil Steril, 1988, 49: 944−955.

[29] DONNEZ J, NISOLLE M. Hysteroscopic lysis of intrauterine adhesions (Asherman syndrome) // DONNEZ J, editor. Atlas of Laser Operative Laparoscopy and Hysteroscopy. New York: Press-Parthenon, 1994: 305−322.

[30] NASR A L, AI-INANY H, THABET S, et al. A clinicohysteroscopic scoring system of intrauterine adhesions. Gynecol Obstet Invest, 2000, 50: 178−181.

[31] ROY K K, NEGI N, SUBBAIAN M, et al. Effectiveness of estrogen in the prevention of intrauterine adhesions after hysteroscopic septal resection: a prospective, randomized study. J Obstet Gynaecol Res, 2014, 40: 1085－1088.

[32] TONGUC E A, VAR T, YILMAZ N, et al. Intrauterine device or estrogen treatment after hysteroscopic uterine septum resection. Int J Gynaecol Obstet, 2010, 109: 226－229.

[33] DI SPIEZIO S A, SPINELLI M, BRAMANTE S, et al. Efficacy of a polyethylene oxide-sodium carboxymethylcellulose gel in prevention of intrauterine adhesions after hysteroscopic surgery. J Minim Invasive Gynecol, 2011, 18: 462－469.

[34] FUCHS N, SMORGICK N, BEN AMI I, et al. Intercoat (Oxiplex/AP gel) for preventing intrauterine adhesions after operative hysteroscopy for suspected retained products of conception: double-blind, prospective, randomized pilot study. J Minim Invasive Gynecol, 2014, 21: 126－130.

[35] GUIDA M, ACUNZO G, DI SPIEZIO S A, et al. Effectiveness of autocrosslinked hyaluronic acid gel in the prevention of intrauterine adhesions after hysteroscopic surgery: a prospective, randomized, controlled study. Hum Reprod, 2004, 19: 1461－1464.

[36] TSAPANOS V S, STATHOPOULOU L P, PAPATHANASSOPOULOU V S, et al. The role of Seprafilm bioresorbable membrane in the prevention and therapy of endometrial synechiae. J Biomed Mater Res, 2002, 63: 10－14.

[37] KIM T, AHN K H, CHOI D S, et al. A randomized, multi-center, clinical trial to assess the efficacy and safety of alginate carboxymethylcellulose hyaluronic acid compared to carboxymethylcellulose hyaluronic acid to prevent postoperative intrauterine adhesion. J Minim Invasive Gynecol, 2012, 19: 731－736.

[38] DE IACO P A, MUZZUPAPA G, BOVICELLI A, et al. Hyaluronan derivative gel (Hyalobarrier gel) in intrauterine adhesion (IUA) prevention after operative hysteroscopy. Ellipse, 2003, 19: 15－18.

[39] MENSITIERI M, AMBROSIO L, NICOLAIS L, et al. Visco-elastic

properties modulation of a novel autocrosslinked hyaluronic acid polymer. J Mater Sci Mater Med, 1996, 7: 695-698.

[40] BEN-AMI I, MELCER Y, SMORGICK N, et al. A comparison of reproductive outcomes following hysteroscopic management versus dilatation and curettage of retained products of conception. Int J Gynaecol Obstet, 2014, 127: 86-89.

[41] FAIVRE E, DEFFIEUX X, MRAZGUIA C, et al. Hysteroscopic management of residual trophoblastic tissue and reproductive outcome: a pilot study. J Minim Invasive Gynecol, 2009, 16: 487-490.

[42] GOLAN A, DISHI M, SHALEV A, et al. Operative hysteroscopy to remove retained products of conception: novel treatment of an old problem. J Minim Invasive Gynecol, 2011, 18: 100-103.

[43] REIN D T, SCHMIDT T, HESS A P, et al. Hysteroscopic management of residual trophoblastic tissue is superior to ultrasound-guided curettage. J Minim Invasive Gynecol, 2011, 18: 774-778.

[44] YANG J H, CHEN M J, CHEN C D, et al. Optimal waiting period for subsequent fertility treatment after various hysteroscopic surgeries. Fertil Steril, 2013, 99: 2092-2096, e3.

[45] TASKIN O, SADIK S, ONOGLU A, et al. Role of endometrial suppression on the frequency of intrauterine adhesions after resectoscopic surgery. J Am Assoc Gynecol Laparosc, 2000, 7: 351-354.

[46] FEDELE L, BIANCHI S, FRONTINO G. Septums and synechiae: approaches to surgical correction. Clin Obstet Gynecol, 2006, 49: 767-788.

[47] MAZZON I, FAVILLI A, COCCO P, et al. Does cold loop hysteroscopic myomectomy reduce intrauterine adhesions: a retrospective study. Fertil Steril, 2014, 101: 294-298, e3.

[48] SHOKEIR T A, FAWZY M, TATONGY M. The nature of intrauterine adhesions following reproductive hysteroscopic surgery as determined by early and late follow-up hysteroscopy: clinical implications. Arch Gynecol Obstet, 2008, 277: 423-427.

[49] SCHENKER J G, MARGALIOTH E J. Intrauterine adhesions: an updated appraisal. Fertil Steril, 1982, 37: 593-610.

[50] ASHERMAN J G. Traumatic intra-uterine adhesions. J Obstet Gynaecol Br Emp, 1950, 57: 892-896.

[51] SUGIMOTO O. Diagnostic and therapeutic hysteroscopy for traumatic intrauterine adhesions. Am J Obstet Gynecol, 1978, 131: 539-547.

[52] DEANS R, ABBOTT J. Review of intrauterine adhesions. J Minim Invasive Gynecol, 2010, 17: 555-569.

[53] CAPELLA-ALLOUC S, MORSAD F, RONGIERES-BERTRAND C, et al. Hysteroscopic treatment of severe Asherman's syndrome and subsequent fertility. Hum Reprod, 1999, 14: 1230-1233.

[54] CHAPMAN R, CHAPMAN K. The value of two stage laser treatment for severe Asherman's syndrome. Br J Obstet Gynaecol, 1996, 103: 1256-1258.

[55] GOLDENBERG M, SCHIFF E, ACHIRON R, et al. Managing residual trophoblastic tissue: hysteroscopy for directing curettage. J Reprod Med, 1997, 42: 26-28.

[56] PABUCCU R, ATAY V, ORHON E, et al. Hysteroscopic treatment of intrauterine adhesions is safe and effective in the restoration of normal menstruation and fertility. Fertil Steril, 1997, 68: 1141-1143.

[57] FERNANDEZ H, GERVAISE A, DE TAYRAC R. Operative hysteroscopy for infertility using normal saline solution and a coaxial bipolar electrode: a pilot study. Hum Reprod, 2000, 15: 1773-1775.

[58] ZIKOPOULOS K. Live delivery rates in subfertile women with Asherman's syndrome after hysteroscopic adhesiolysis using the resectoscope or the Versapoint system. Reprod Biomed Online, 2004, 8: 720-725.

[59] TOUBOUL C, FERNANDEZ H, DEFFIEUX X, et al. Uterine synechiae after bipolar hysteroscopic resection of submucosal myomas in patients with infertility. Fertil Steril, 2009, 92: 1690-1693.

[60] NEWTON J R, MACKENZIE W E, EMENS M J, et al. Division of

uterine adhesions (Asherman's syndrome) with the Nd-YAG laser. Br J Obstet Gynaecol, 1989, 96: 102—104.

[61] DUFFY S, REID P, SHARP F. In vivo studies of uterine electrosurgery. Br J Obstet Gynaecol, 1992, 99: 579—582.

[62] ROGE P, D'ERCOLE C, CRAVELLO L, et al. Hysteroscopic management of uterine synechiae: a series of 102 observations. Eur J Obstet Gynecol Reprod Biol, 1996, 65: 189—193.

[63] CARARACH M, PANELLA J, UBEDA A, et al. Hysteroscopic incision of the septate uterus: scissors versus resectoscope. Hum Reprod, 1994, 9: 87—89.

[64] BROOME J D, VANCAILLIE T. Fluoroscopically guided hysteroscopic division of adhesions in severe Asherman syndrome. Obstet Gynecol, 1999, 93: 1041—1043.

[65] THOMSON A J, ABBOTT J A, KINGSTON A, et al. Fluoroscopically guided synechiolysis for patients with Asherman's syndrome: menstrual and fertility outcomes. Fertil Steril, 2007, 87: 405—410.

[66] BOUGIE O, LORTIE K, SHENASSA H, et al. Treatment of Asherman's syndrome in an outpatient hysteroscopy setting. J Minim Invasive Gynecol, 2015, 22: 446—450.

[67] PROTOPAPAS A, SHUSHAN A, MAGOS A. Myometrial scoring: a new technique for the management of severe Asherman's syndrome. Fertil Steril, 1998, 69: 860—864.

[68] HANSTEDE M M, VAN DER MEIJ E, GOEDEMANS L, et al. Results of centralized Asherman surgery, 2003—2013. Fertil Steril, 2015, 104: 1561—1568.

[69] KARANDE V, LEVRANT S, HOXSEY R, et al. Lysis of intrauterine adhesions using gynecoradiologic techniques. Fertil Steril, 1997, 68: 658—662.

[70] BELLINGHAM F R. Intrauterine adhesions: hysteroscopic lysis and adjunctive methods. Aust N Z J Obstet Gynaecol, 1996, 36: 171—174.

[71] KRESOWIK J D, SYROP C H, VAN VOORHIS B J, et al. Ultrasound is the optimal choice for guidance in difficult hysteroscopy. Ultrasound Obstet Gynecol, 2012, 39: 715−718.

[72] MCCOMB P F, WAGNER B L. Simplified therapy for Asherman's syndrome. Fertil Steril, 1997, 68: 1047−1050.

[73] FEDELE L, VERCELLINI P, VIEZZOLI T, et al. Intrauterine adhesions: current diagnostic and therapeutic trends. Acta Eur Fertil, 1986, 17: 31−37.

[74] PREUTTHIPAN S, LINASMITA V. A prospective comparative study between hysterosalpingography and hysteroscopy in the detection of intrauterine pathology in patients with infertility. J Obstet Gynaecol Res, 2003, 29: 33−37.

[75] SIEGLER A M, VALLE R F. Therapeutic hysteroscopic procedures. Fertil Steril, 1988, 50: 685−701.

[76] YANG J H, CHEN C D, CHEN S U, et al. The influence of the location and extent of intrauterine adhesions on recurrence after hysteroscopic adhesiolysis. Br J Obstet Gynaecol, 2016, 123: 618−623.

[77] PABUCCU R, ONALAN G, KAYA C, et al. Efficiency and pregnancy outcome of serial intrauterine device-guided hysteroscopic adhesiolysis of intrauterine synechiae. Fertil Steril, 2008, 90: 1973−1977.

[78] VESCE F, JORIZZO G, BIANCIOTTO A, et al. Use of the copper intrauterine device in the management of secondary amenorrhea. Fertil Steril, 2000, 73: 162−165.

[79] MARCH C M, ISRAEL R. Gestational outcomes following hysteroscopic lysis of adhesions. Fertil Steril, 1981, 36: 455−459.

[80] LIN X N, ZHOU F, WEI M L, et al. Randomized, controlled trial comparing the efficacy of intrauterine balloon and intrauterine contraceptive device in the prevention of adhesion reformation after hysteroscopic adhesiolysis. Fertil Steril, 2015, 104: 235−240.

[81] SANFILIPPO J S, FITZGERALD M R, BADAWY S Z, et al.

Asherman's syndrome: a comparison of therapeutic methods. J Reprod Med, 1982, 27: 328—330.

[82] ORHUE A A, AZIKEN M E, IGBEFOH J O. A comparison of two adjunctive treatments for intrauterine adhesions following lysis. Int J Gynaecol Obstet, 2003, 82: 49—56.

[83] AMER M I, ABD-EL-MAEBOUD K H. Amnion graft following hysteroscopic lysis of intrauterine adhesions. J Obstet Gynaecol Res, 2006, 32: 559—566.

[84] YASMIN H, NASIR A, NOORANI K J. Hystroscopic management of Asherman syndrome. J Pak Med Assoc, 2007, 57: 553—555.

[85] AMER M I, ABD-EL-MAEBOUD K H, et al. Human amnion as a temporary biologic barrier after hysteroscopic lysis of severe intrauterine adhesions: pilot study. J Minim Invasive Gynecol, 2010, 17: 605—611.

[86] LIN Y H, JANG T N, WANG J L, et al. Bacterial colonization with balloon uterine stent placement in the uterus for 30 days: a randomized controlled clinical trial. Fertil Steril, 2015, 103: 513—518, e2.

[87] ACUNZO G, GUIDA M, PELLICANO M, et al. Effectiveness of auto-cross-linked hyaluronic acid gel in the prevention of intrauterine adhesions after hysteroscopic adhesiolysis: a prospective, randomized, controlled study. Hum Reprod, 2003, 18: 1918—1921.

[88] LIN X, WEI M, LI T C, et al. A comparison of intrauterine balloon, intrauterine contraceptive device and hyaluronic acid gel in the prevention of adhesion reformation following hysteroscopic surgery for Asherman syndrome: a cohort study. Eur J Obstet Gynecol Reprod Biol, 2013, 170: 512—516.

[89] HUBERLANT S, FERNANDEZ H, VIEILLE P, et al. Application of a hyaluronic acid gel after intrauterine surgery may improve spontaneous fertility: a randomized controlled trial in New Zealand White rabbits. PLoS One, 2015, 10: e0125610.

[90] HSIEH Y Y, TSAI H D, CHANG C C, et al. Low dose aspirin for infertile women with thin endometrium receiving intrauterine insemination: a pro-

spective, randomized study. J Assist Reprod Genet, 2000, 17: 174—177.

[91] HURST B S, BHOJWANI J T, MARSHBURN P B, et al. Low-dose aspirin does not improve ovarian stimulation, endometrial response, or pregnancy rates for in vitro fertilization. J Exp Clin Assist Reprod, 2005, 31: 8—12.

[92] SHER G, FISCH J D. Effect of vaginal sildenafil on the outcome of in vitro fertilization (IVF) after multiple IVF failures attributed to poor endo-metrial development. Fertil Steril, 2002, 78: 1073—1076.

[93] ZACKRISSON U, BRANNSTROM M, GRANBERG S, et al. Acute effects of a transdermal nitric oxide donor on perifollicular and intrauterine blood flow. Ultrasound Obstet Gynecol, 1998, 12: 50—55.

[94] ZINGER M, LIU J H, THOMAS M A. Successful use of vaginal sildenafil citrate in two infertility patients with Asherman's syndrome. J Womens Health, 2006, 15: 442—444.

[95] ACOG Committee on Practice Bulletins. ACOG Practice Bulletin No. 74: Antibiotic prophylaxis for gynecologic procedures. Obstet Gynecol, 2006, 108: 225—234.

[96] GARGETT C E, YE L. Endometrial reconstruction from stem cells. Fertil Steril, 2012, 98: 11—20.

[97] ALAWADHI F, DU H, CAKMAK H, et al. Bone Marrow-Derived Stem Cell (BMDSC) transplantation improves fertility in a murine model of Asherman's syndrome. PLoS One, 2014, 9: e96662.

[98] KILIC S, YUKSEL B, PINARLI F, et al. Effect of stem cell application on Asherman syndrome, an experimental rat model. J Assist Reprod Genet, 2014, 31: 975—982.

[99] KURAMOTO G, TAKAGI S, ISHITANI K, et al. Preventive effect of oral mucosal epithelial cell sheets on intrauterine adhesions. Hum Reprod, 2015, 30: 406—416.

[100] SANTAMARIA X, CABANILLAS S, CERVELLO I, et al. Autologous cell therapy with CD1331 bone marrow-derived stem cells for refractory Asherman's syndrome and endometrial atrophy: a pilot cohort study. Hum Re-

prod, 2016, 31: 1087—1096.

[101] MARCH C M. Management of Asherman's syndrome. Reprod Biomed Online, 2011, 23: 63—76.

[102] XIAO S, WAN Y, XUE M, et al. Etiology, treatment, and reproductive prognosis of women with moderate-to-severe intrauterine adhesions. Int J Gynaecol Obstet, 2014, 125: 121—124.

[103] SONG D, LIU Y, XIAO Y, et al. A matched cohort study comparing the outcome of intrauterine adhesiolysis for Asherman's syndrome after uterine artery embolization or surgical trauma. J Minim Invasive Gynecol, 2014, 21: 1022—1028.

[104] FUGLSANG J. Later reproductive health after B-Lynch sutures: a follow-up study after 10 years' clinical use of the B-Lynch suture. Fertil Steril, 2014, 101: 1194—1199.

[105] RATHAT G, DO TRINH P, MERCIER G, et al. Synechia after uterine compression sutures. Fertil Steril, 2011, 95: 405—409.

[106] BOSTEELS J, WEYERS S, MOL B W, et al. Anti-adhesion barrier gels following operative hysteroscopy for treating female infertility: a systematic review and meta-analysis. Gynecol Surg, 2014, 11: 113—127.

AAGL practice report:

practice guidelines on intrauterine adhesions developed in collaboration with the European Society of Gynaecological Endoscopy (ESGE)

What is new in this report?

Substantial progress has been made since publishing previous practice guidelines on intrauterine adhesions (IUAs)[1]. Large-scale series, although retrospective, have reported clinical outcomes. Randomized controlled trials (RCTs) have investigated both primary and secondary adhesion prevention including solid and semi-solid barriers, although individual surgical techniques have not been rigorously studied. Recent human studies documenting successful pregnancy outcomes for bone marrow-derived stem cell (BMDSC) treatments following intermittent hysteroscopy are reported. This may provide a new avenue for research, although high quality data demonstrating efficacy are required before being introduced as a treatment option for women with symptomatic IUAs (Asherman syndrome).

In order to encourage their wide dissemination, these guidelines are freely accessible on the GYNS and JMIG websites.

Background

Intrauterine adhesions have been recognized as a cause of secondary amenorrhea since the end of the nineteenth century[2], and in the mid-twentieth century, Asherman further described the eponymous condition occurring after pregnancy[3, 4]. The terms "Asherman syndrome" and IUAs are often used interchangeably, although the syndrome requires the constellation of signs and symptoms (in this case, pain, menstrual disturbance, and subfertility in any combination) related to the presence of IUAs[3, 4]. The presence of IUAs in the absence of symptoms may be best referred to as asymptomatic IUAs and are of questionable clinical significance. In these guidelines, we use the term "IUAs" specifying whether or not they are associated with clinical symptoms.

Identification and assessment of evidence

The AAGL Practice Guidelines were produced by searching electronic databases including MEDLINE, PubMed, CINAHL, the Cochrane Library (including the Cochrane Database of Systematic Reviews), Current Contents, and EMBASE for all articles related to IUAs up to and including week 4 of April 2016. The MeSH (in MEDLARS) terms included all subheadings, and keywords included Asherman syndrome; Intrauterine adhesions; Intrauterine septum and synechiae; Hysteroscopic lysis of adhesions; Hysteroscopic synechiolysis; Hysteroscopy and adhesion and Obstetric outcomes following intrauterine surgery.

The search was not restricted to English language literature; committee members fluent in languages other than English reviewed relevant articles and provided the committee with relative information translated into English. All published works were included from the electronic database searches, and relevant articles not available in electronic sources (e. g. , published before the beginning of electronic database commencement) were cross-referenced from hand-searched bibliographies and included in the literature review. When necessary, authors were contacted directly for clarification of published data. All studies were assessed for methodological rigor and graded according to the US Preventive Services Task Force classification system outlined in the previous practice guidelines on IUAs[1]. Recommendations were based on the best available evidence, where possible, and where such evidence was not available, upon consensus of the expert panel.

Diagnosis

In women with suspected Asherman syndrome, physical examination frequently fails to reveal abnormalities[5, 6]. Blind, transcervical uterine sounding may reveal cervical obstruction at or near the level of the internal os[6]; however, adhesions higher in the cavity or more laterally may not be demonstrated in this manner. Hysteroscopy has been established as the criterion standard for diagnosis of IUAs[7]. Compared with radiologic investigations, and provided the endometrial cavity is accessible, hysteroscopy more accurately confirms the presence, extent, and morphological characteristics of adhesions and the quality of the endometrium. It provides a real-time view of the cavity, enabling accurate description of location and degree of adhesions, classification, and concurrent treatment of IUAs[8].

Hysterosalpingography (HSG) using contrast dye has a sensitivity of 75 to 81%, specificity of 80%, and positive predictive value of 50% compared with hysteroscopy for diagnosis of IUAs[9, 10]. The high false-positive rate (up to 39%)[11] limits its use, and it does not detect endometrial fibrosis[4] or the nature and extent of IUAs[12], and therefore, use should be confined to that of a screening test.

Sonohysterography [SHG; also called saline infusion sonography (SIS) or gel infusion sonography (GIS)] was found to be as effective as HSG, with both reported to have a sensitivity of 75% and positive predictive value of 43% for SHG or SIS/GIS and 50% for HSG, compared with hysteroscopy[10, 13]. Imaging techniques do appear to be hierarchical with two-dimensional gray-scale transvaginal ultrasonography having a sensitivity of 52% and specificity of 11% compared with hysteroscopy[13]. Three-dimensional (3D) ultrasonography may be more helpful in the evaluation of IUAs, with sensitivity reported to be 87% and specificity of 45% when compared with 3D SHG (although this study did not compare with hysteroscopy)[14]. 3D SHG has a high specificity of 87% although a lower sensitivity of 70% when compared with the standard, hysteroscopy[15].

Newer techniques currently being investigated include power Doppler sonography where studies suggest high resistance flows that are associated with poorer obstetric outcomes[16], and the addition of contrast color power angiography to 3D ultrasonography may have a role in both initial assessment and prognosis for women with Asherman syndrome[17]. Initial assessments of magnetic resonance imaging (MRI) for the diagnosis of IUAs show few advantages over less costly alternatives[18-20], with more recent assessment of gadolinium-enhanced images showing some promise[21, 22]. None of these techniques have been fully evaluated or can be recommended for routine practice until further research is undertaken[23].

Guidelines for diagnosis of intrauterine adhesions

1. Hysteroscopy is the most accurate method for diagnosis of IUAs and should be the investigation of choice when available. Level B.

2. If hysteroscopy is not available, HSG and SHG are reasonable alternatives. Level B.

3. Magnetic resonance imaging should not be used for diagnosis of IUAs outside of clinical research studies. Level C.

Classification

Classification of IUAs is useful because prognosis is related to the severity of disease[8]. A number of classification systems have been proposed for IUAs, each of which includes hysteroscopy to determine the characteristics of adhesions[24]. To date, there are no data from any comparative analysis of these classification systems. Table 1 gives the available classification systems and their key features.

Table 1　Classification of intrauterine adhesions

Source	Summary of classification
March et al. [7]	Adhesions classified as minimal, moderate, or severe based on hysteroscopic assessment of the degree of uterine cavity involvement.
Hamou et al. [25]	Adhesions classified as isthmic, marginal, central, or severe according to hysteroscopic assessment.
Valle and Sciarra[26]	Adhesions classified as mild, moderate, or severe according to hysteroscopic assessment and extent of occlusion (partial or total) at HSG.
European Society for Hysteroscopy[27]	Complex system classifies IUAs as grades I through IV with several subtypes and incorporates a combination of hysteroscopic and HSG findings and clinical symptoms.
American Fertility Society[28]	Complex scored system of mild, moderate, or severe IUAs based on extent of endometrial cavity obliteration, appearance of adhesions, and patient menstrual characteristics based on hysteroscopic or HSG assessment.
Donnez and Nisolle[29]	Adhesions classified into six grades on the basis of location, with postoperative pregnancy rate the primary driver. Hysteroscopy or HSG are used for assessment.
Nasr et al. [30]	Complex system creates a prognostic score by incorporating menstrual and obstetric history with IUA findings at hysteroscopic assessment.

Guidelines for classification of intrauterine adhesions

1. Intrauterine adhesions should be classified as prognosis is correlated with severity of adhesions. Level B.

2. The various classification systems make comparison between studies diffi-

cult to interpret. This may reflect inherent deficiencies in each of the classification systems. Consequently, it is currently not possible to endorse any specific system. Level C.

Primary prevention

There are eight RCTs reporting outcomes on methods for primary prevention of IUAs following surgical procedures[31-38]. The first RCT evaluated the value of using oral estrogen postoperatively following hysteroscopic septoplasty and reported no significant difference of de novo adhesion formation[31]. At secondlook hysteroscopy, there were no adhesions in 42 women assigned to take 2 mg of estradiol valerate per day for 30 days postoperatively while synechiae were seen in 3 of 43 women (7%) in the placebo group. There was no difference in subsequent pregnancy rates (37% estrogen group vs 41% placebo group) at up to 2 years follow-up. Similar data were reported in a second RCT of 100 women having hysteroscopic septoplasty whose postoperative management included (1) no treatment, (2) the use of estrogen alone, (3) estrogens and a copper-containing intrauterine device (IUD), or (4) copper-containing IUD alone[32]. There was no reported difference in the rate of postoperative de novo adhesion formation assessed hysteroscopically, and there were no differences in pregnancy outcomes.

Six RCTs have assessed the role of semi-solid (gel) adhesion barriers used postoperatively[33-38] as they may be suitable for preventing IUAs owing to high sensitivity and prolonged time on an injured surface such as the postoperative endometrium[39]. These studies randomized women and compared polyethylene oxide-sodium carboxymethylcellulose gel and hyaluronic acid derivatives against control groups or against each other. For two of these studies, procedures unrelated to pregnancy were examined and reported a significant reduction in de novo adhesion formation when barriers were used compared with controls (3/55 [5%] vs 12/55 [22%][33] and 7/67 [10%] vs 17/65 [26%][35]; $P<0.05$ for both studies). The third of these studies did not report a reduction in de novo adhesion formation in blinded follow-up with 13/18 (72%) treated women versus 15/22 (68%) women in the control group with no adhesions at 9 weeks follow-up[38].

Adhesions were more likely to be severe in the control group, although not statistically significant. Unfortunately, none of these studies report data on subsequent pregnancy.

The sixth of these RCTs examined primary prevention in women following hysteroscopic removal of retained products of conception and demonstrated no statistical difference for rate of moderate to severe adhesions at 6 to 8 weeks following the procedure (1 woman [4%] receiving barrier vs 3 [14%] controls; P =0. 3) or subsequent pregnancy (7 women [27%] in the barrier group vs 3 [14%] controls P=0. 5) in the 20-month mean follow-up period[34]. The seventh RCT followed 150 women who underwent suction curettage after incomplete, missed, or recurrent miscarriage[36]. Fifty women were randomized to receive an adhesion barrier, and 100 patients served as the control group. In the adhesion barrier group, 32 of 32 patients (100%) became pregnant within 8 months following the procedure compared with 34 of 56 patients (54%) in the control group. Adhesions were found in 1 of 10 women (10%) receiving treatment compared with 7 of 14 (50%) in the control group who had not become pregnant. No adverse events were reported in the treatment group.

In the final RCT studying primary prevention, alginate carboxymethylcellulose hyaluronic acid was compared with carboxycellulose hyaluronic acid in 187 women having various types of hysteroscopic surgery and showed no difference in adhesion severity between the two groups overall, although the alginate carboxymethylcellulose hyaluronic acid was reported to be a better primary prevention product (P=0. 02)[37].

The surgical approach may impact subsequent adhesion formation with retrospective data reporting that a hysteroscopic approach may have benefit over blind curettage[40-42] or ultrasound-guided curettage[43]. Whereas these studies also report an earlier time to next pregnancy, their methodological limitations indicate the need for further evaluation. The type of hysteroscopic procedure being performed may also impact healing and determine subsequent formation of IUAs. Prospective evaluations of hysteroscopic procedures report that the endometrium heals fastest with polypectomy and slowest following septoplasty[44]. The lowest incidence of adhesion formation follows polypectomy with the highest rate of adhesion formation following multiple fibroid resection[45]. The mode of hysteroscopic surgery may be important with avoidance of electrosurgery for myomectomy where adhesions have been documented adjacent to the excised pathology[46-48]. More recently, a large retrospective cohort study has been published reporting lower rates (4%) of IUAs with a hysteroscopic myomectomy technique that combines minimal use of radio frequency electrical energy with cold loop dissection[47].

Guidelines for primary prevention of intrauterine adhesions

1. The risk for de novo adhesions during hysteroscopic surgery is impacted by the type of procedure performed with those confined to the endometrium (polypectomy) having the lowest risk and those entering the myometrium or involving opposing surfaces a higher risk. Level B

2. The method of pathology removal may impact the risk of de novo adhesions. The risk appears to be greater when electrosurgery is used in the nongravid uterus and for blind versus vision-guided removal in the gravid uterus. Level C

3. The application of an adhesion barrier following surgery that may lead to endometrial damage significantly reduces the development of IUAs in the short term, although limited fertility data are available following this intervention. Level A

Management of intrauterine adhesions

As IUAs are not life-threatening, treatment should be considered only when there are signs or symptoms of pain, infertility, recurrent pregnancy loss, or menstrual abnormalities including hematometra. Surgery has been the criterion standard in the management of Asherman syndrome; however, there are no RCTs comparing surgical intervention and expectant management nor are there RCTs comparing different methods of surgical interventions for Asherman syndrome. The primary objective of any intervention is to restore the normal volume and shape of the endometrial cavity and cervical canal and to facilitate communication between the cavity and both the cervical canal and fallopian tubes. This will allow both normal menstrual flow and adequate sperm transportation for fertilization and implantation to occur.

Expectant management

The limited data supporting a role for expectant management, published in 1982, demonstrated resumption of menstruation in as many as 78% within 7 years from diagnosis of IUAs and pregnancy in 45.5% of women[49].

Cervical probing

Cervical stenosis without damage to the uterine cavity or endometrium has been treated using cervical probing with or without ultrasound guidance[50]. All available data were accrued before the advent of hysteroscopically directed adhesiolysis, and uterine perforation has been reported after blind cervical probing. Consequently, this technique currently has a limited role.

Dilation and curettage

Dilation and curettage was the primary mode of management before the widespread use of hysteroscopy, and reported results included return to normal menses in 1049 of 1250 women (84%), conception in 540 of 1052 women (51%), miscarriages in 142 of 559 pregnancies (25%), term delivery in 306 of 559 pregnancies (55%), premature delivery in 50 of 559 pregnancies (9%), and complicated by placenta accreta in 42 of 559 pregnancies (8%)[49]. The severity of adhesions in this group is unknown, though most were likely mild. With the availability of hysteroscopy, dilation and curettage should not be performed as accurate diagnosis and classification are not possible and further damage to the endometrium may occur.

Hysteroscopy

Hysteroscopic treatment enables lysis of IUAs under direct vision and with magnification. The uterine distention required for hysteroscopy may itself lyse mild adhesions, and blunt dissection may be performed using only the tip of the hysteroscope[51]. The more lateral the adhesions and the greater their density, the more difficult the dissection and the greater the risk of complications such as uterine perforation[4, 52]. Monopolar[26, 53-56] and bipolar[57-59] electrosurgical instruments and the Nd-YAG laser[26, 54, 60] have been described as techniques used to lyse adhesions under direct vision, with the advantages of precise cutting and good hemostasis. Disadvantages include potential visceral damage if uterine perforation occurs[8], further endometrial damage predisposing to recurrence of IUAs[61, 62], cost, and the degree of cervical dilation required to accommodate operative instruments. None of these techniques has been compared with any other; consequently, there is no available evidence that one method is superior to any other. Indirect evidence exists to avoid electrosurgery during adhesiolysis owing to the potential risk for further endometrial damage[63]. Mechanical division of adhesions by scissors[7, 26] and needle[64, 65] are described as modes of surgical treatment. Surgical treatment may also take place in an office or outpatient setting with outcomes similar to those in an inpatient setting[66].

Other hysteroscopic techniques

Techniques have been described for the treatment of severe cohesive IUAs when typical hysteroscopically directed techniques are not possible or safe. Myometrial scoring has been effective for the creation of a uterine cavity in women with severe IUAs. In this technique, six to eight 4-mm-deep incisions are created in the myometrium using electrosurgery with a Collins knife electrode from the fundus to the cervix. These incisions enable widening of the uterine cavity. Anatomic success has been reported in 71% of patients in one small series[67], and 51.6% in another[53], with pregnancy achieved in 3 of 7 women in the small series (42.9%) and 12 of 31 women in the other (38.7%).

Additional guiding techniques for hysteroscopy

Fluoroscopically guided blunt dissection of severe adhesions has been described using a hysteroscopically directed Tuohy needle under image intensifier control with the patient under general anesthesia[64]. This technique is costly, exposes the patient to ionizing radiation, and is technically challenging. Its advantages include use of a narrow hysteroscope, reduced risk of uterine perforation, and reduced risk of visceral damage should perforation occur, because no energy source is applied[65, 68]. A similar technique is described in an ambulatory setting using local anesthesia[69], with described success in mild adhesions only.

Transabdominal ultrasound has been described as a technique to guide hysteroscopic division of IUAs[4, 62, 67, 70, 71]. Advantages of the technique include the availability of ultrasound and its noninvasive nature; however, uterine perforation has been reported in as many as 5% of cases[58, 67, 72]. Laparoscopic guidance is reported to aid hysteroscopically directed division of severe IUAs and enable concurrent inspection of the pelvic organs[58, 67, 72].

Another approach described for treatment of IUAs with cavity obliteration is the use of a cervical dilator sequentially directed from the cervical canal toward the two ostia, creating two lateral landmarks and a central fibrous septum, which is then divided transcervically with a hysteroscopic technique under laparoscopic guidance. A small series of six women has been reported, with uterine perforation in two women and substantial hemorrhage in another[72]. The increased cost and potential morbidity associated with laparoscopy must be considered, and despite improved fertility, with such limited data and high morbidity, this technique cannot be recommended.

Nonhysteroscopic methods of treating intrauterine adhesions

Laparotomy, hysterotomy, and subsequent blunt dissection through adhesions using a finger or curette have been traditional treatments for severe IUAs[6, 50, 58, 62]. A review of 31 cases and case series treated using this approach reported conception in 16 of 31 women (52%), with live births in 11 (38%) including 8 (26%) who delivered at term. Of the 16 women who conceived, placenta accreta complicated the pregnancy in 5 (31%)[49]. In contemporary practice, this technique is rarely used and is reserved only for severe cases in which other techniques are not practical or possible[73].

Guidelines for the surgical management of intrauterine adhesions

1. Hysteroscopic lysis of adhesions by direct vision and a tool for adhesiolysis is the recommended approach for symptomatic IUAs. Level B

2. There is no evidence to support the use of blind cervical probing. Level C.

3. There is no evidence to support the use of blind dilation and curettage. Level C.

4. For women with IUAs who do not wish any intervention but still want to conceive, expectant management may result in subsequent pregnancy; however, the time interval may be prolonged. Level C.

5. Adjunctive interventions to aid adhesiolysis include ultrasound, fluoroscopy, and laparoscopy. There are no data to suggest that these prevent perforation or improve surgical outcomes and are likely dependent on clinical skills and availability. However, when such an approach is used in appropriately selected patients, it may minimize the consequences if perforation occurs. Level B

6. In the presence of extensive or dense adhesions, treatment should be performed by an expert hysteroscopist familiar with at least one of the methods described. Level C.

Secondary prevention

Having undertaken surgical adhesiolysis, it is recognized that recurrence is common and may occur in 30 to 66% of women treated for IUAs[26, 53, 74—76]. Methods to reduce recurrence have been assessed by an increasing number of randomized trials using a variety of solid and semi-solid (gel) barriers. Traditional solid barrier techniques of separating the uterine walls following adhesiolysis include the use of an IUD, amnion graft, or stent, typically comprising an intrauterine catheter with an inflatable balloon tip. The use of gels such as hyaluronic acid and polyethylene oxide-sodium carboxymethylcellulose has also been subjected to more stringent investigation, and in total, five RCTs are currently evaluating outcomes for secondary prevention strategies.

Solid barriers

Insertion of an IUD to separate the endometrial layers after lysis of IUAs has been described for many years[7, 49, 77]. Copper-containing and T-shaped IUDs cannot be recommended because of their inflammation-provoking properties[78] and small surface area[79], respectively. An inert loop IUD (e. g. , Lippes loop) is considered the IUD of choice when treating IUAs[4], although it is no longer available in many geographic areas. In a prospective comparative study of 71 women, the use of second-look hysteroscopy was evaluated following insertion of a Lippes loop and estrogen and progestin treatment for 2 months[77]. Women in group 1 underwent early repeat hysteroscopy at 1 week and then reassessment following removal of the IUD at 2 months following index procedure. Group 2 did not have an early repeat hysteroscopy. There was no difference in pregnancy rates or live births and no comparison to women not having an IUD. A randomized study compared an IUD in 80 women with an intrauterine balloon stent in 82 women, each placed for 1 week following hysteroscopic treatment of adhesions[80]. The outcome measure was hysteroscopically rated adhesion score at 1 to 2 months following index treatment, and this study reported no difference in adhesion reformation rate between the balloon group (30%) and the IUD group (35%). This study did not report pregnancy outcomes or compare adhesions in women not receiving any postoperative intervention. In a small nonrandomized study, postoperative IUD plus hormone therapy was compared with hormone therapy alone, with no significant difference reported for adhesion reformation[81]. The risk of infection when an IUD is introduced into the uterus immediately after adhesiolysis is estimated to be 8%[82], and perforation of the uterus during IUD insertion has been reported[82].

The use of a Foley catheter for 3 to 10 days following surgical lysis of IUAs is similarly reported to act as a physical intrauterine barrier[7, 50, 56, 69, 83, 84]. A nonrandomized study compared the use of an inflated pediatric Foley catheter in place for 10 days postoperatively in 59 patients with that of an IUD in situ for 3 months in 51 patients[82]. There were fewer infections in the Foley group and a lower recurrence rate of IUAs as assessed using HSG[82]. Although amenorrhea continued in 19% of women in the Foley group and 38% in the IUD group, the fertility rate was relatively low in both groups: 20 of 59 (34%) and 14 of 51 (28%), respectively. In a study of 25 women with moderate to severe IUAs, use of a fresh amnion graft over an inflated Foley catheter prevented recurrence of IUAs in 52% of women, although follow-up fertility data and complications were not reported[83].

A three-armed pilot RCT assessed fresh amnion versus dried amnion grafts versus intrauterine balloon alone[85]. Forty-five women were randomized (15 in each group), and each underwent diagnostic hysteroscopy 2 to 4 months following treatment. Amnion grafts reduced adhesions significantly more than the balloon alone ($P<0.003$), and fresh amnion was superior to dried amnion ($P<0.05$). Ten women (23%) conceived with six (60%) having a miscarriage.

The issue of infection with the insertion of an intrauterine stent has been assessed in an RCT of 60 women (30 women randomized to receive the stent; 30 women as a control)[86]. Hysteroscopic procedures were performed, and the outcome measure was bacterial colonization 30 days after the procedure. There was no difference between control (13 and 33%) and stent (10 and 30%) for bacterial colonization rates before and after stent placement suggesting that infection risk is not substantially impacted by the use of an intrauterine stent.

Semi-solid barriers

A number of gel adhesion barriers are reported to be successful at reducing the risk of adhesion recurrence after surgical treatment of IUAs[35, 36, 87]. Auto-cross-linked hyaluronic acid gel may be suitable for preventing IUAs because of high sensitivity and prolonged time on an injured surface such as the postoperative endometrium[39]. An RCT of 84 women compared auto-cross-linked hyaluronic acid gel with no therapy after surgical treatment of IUAs. Postoperative ultrasound studies demonstrated that the walls of the uterine cavity remained separated for at least 72 h in the barrier group. At second-look hysteroscopy 3 months after the procedure, IUAs were significantly reduced in women receiving the adhesion barrier compared with the control group (6 of 43 [14%] vs 13 of 41 [32%]; $P<0.05$)[87]. Fertility data were not reported in this study.

A retrospective cohort study compared balloon catheter, IUD, hyaluronic gel, and control groups for the reduction of IUAs and found the reduction to be significantly greater in the balloon group compared with the other three groups ($P<0.001$). The reduction of IUAs in the IUD group was greater than those of the gel group ($P<0.001$) and control groups ($P<0.001$), and the reduction in the gel group was not different than the control group[88].

Data from randomized animal studies have reported an increase in pregnancy rate when hyaluronic acid barriers are used following induced IUAs[89]. It remains to be seen if the decrease in adhesion reformation rate extrapolates into increased subsequent pregnancy success following treatment with a gel barrier.

Hormonal treatments

Postoperative treatment with estrogen therapy (a daily oral dose of 2.5 mg conjugated equine estrogen with or without opposing progestin for 2 or 3 cycles)[24, 64, 65, 73] has been described after surgical treatment of IUAs. No comparative studies have been performed to investigate dosage, administration, or combination of hormones. One nonrandomized study reported that hormone treatment alone is as effective as hormone treatment and IUD in combination[81].

Techniques to increase vascular flow to endometrium

Various studies have described use of medications such as aspirin, nitroglycerine, and sildenafil citrate to increase vascular perfusion to the endometrium[90—93] and enable pregnancy[94]. However, the number of women treated using these therapies remains small, and because all such treatment is off-label, these medications cannot be endorsed outside of rigorous research protocols.

Antibiotic therapy

There are no data to support the routine use of antibiotic therapy before, during, or after surgical treatment of IUAs. The American College of Obstetricians and Gynecologists guidelines for antibiotic use in gynecologic procedures do not recommend antibiotic use for diagnostic or operative hysteroscopy[95]. There is, however, a theoretic risk of secondary infection, and it has been proposed that infection may be a primary cause of IUAs. This has led many surgeons to treat women undergoing surgical lysis of IUAs with preoperative or intraoperative antibiotic therapy, and some continue with postoperative antibiotic therapy; however, at this time, there is no evidence to support or refute the use of antibiotic therapy.

Stem cell treatments for intrauterine adhesions

The use of human stem cell treatments for the reconstruction of the endometrium following substantial damage and IUA formation has been hypothesized for some time[96], with studies from animal models showing substantial promise in this area of medical treatment[97-99]. From the first prospective series in humans, 16 women with substantial hysteroscopically confirmed IUAs were treated by uterine intravascular infusions of BMDSC[100]. Clinical, hysteroscopic, and fertility data are reported subsequently, with menstrual function returning to normal within 6 months of BMDSC infusion and three spontaneous pregnancies and seven pregnancies following in vitro fertilization recorded. These initial data from a human series represent the first adjunct treatment of this type for the treatment of Asherman syndrome with successful menstrual and fertility outcomes. It is imperative that wellconducted RCTs are performed to establish the role of BMDSC treatment in addition to or independent of surgical treatments before it is made available to women.

Guidelines for secondary prevention of intrauterine adhesions

1. The use of an IUD, stent, or catheter appears to reduce the rate of postoperative adhesion reformation. There are limited data regarding subsequent fertility outcomes when these barriers are used. Grade A

2. The risk of infection appears to be minimal when a solid barrier is used compared with no treatment. Grade A

3. There is no evidence to support or refute the use of preoperative, intraoperative, or postoperative antibiotic therapy in surgical treatment of IUAs. Grade C

4. If an IUD is used postoperatively, it should be inert and have a large surface area such as a Lippes loop. Intrauterine devices that contain progestin or copper should not be used after surgical division of IUAs. Grade C

5. Semi-solid barriers such as hyaluronic acid and auto-cross-linked hyaluronic acid gel reduce adhesion reformation. At this time, their effect on posttreatment pregnancy rates is unknown. Grade A

6. Following hysteroscopic-directed adhesiolysis, postoperative hormone treatment using estrogen, with or without progestin, may reduce recurrence of IUAs. Grade B

7. The role of medications designed as adjuvants to improve vascular flow to the endometrium has not been established. Consequently, they should not be used outside of rigorous research protocols. Grade C

8. Stem cell treatment may ultimately provide an effective adjuvant approach to the treatment of Asherman syndrome; however, evidence is very limited and this treatment should not be offered outside of rigorous research protocols. Grade C

Postoperative assessment

The recurrence rate is as high as one in three women with mild to moderate IUAs[26, 74, 75] and two of three with severe IUAs[53, 76]. Consequently, and regardless of the surgical intervention used, reassessment of the uterine cavity is considered worthwhile, usually after two to three menstrual cycles following surgery[53]. Ambulatory methods include office hysteroscopy and HSG, with recurrence of more than mild IUAs likely requiring anesthetic and division. Early reintervention with assessment a few weeks after hysteroscopy rather than several months has been suggested in randomized[75] and retrospective studies[99, 100] to both assess and treat recurrence.

Guidelines for postoperative assessment after treatment of intrauterine adhesions

1. Follow-up assessment of the uterine cavity after treatment of IUAs is recommended, preferably with hysteroscopy. Grade B

Outcomes

The outcome measures for treating symptomatic IUAs include adhesion scores, menstrual data, pregnancy rates, and clinical outcomes. The available published evidence is principally retrospective, with a few large-scale data sets now available. The best reported fertility outcome is from a single surgeon who reports a live birth in 674/807 (84%) women followed, although the total number of treated women in this analysis is unclear[101]. A retrospective cohort of 683 women with moderate to severe adhesions treated surgically with postoperative adjuvants including one or a combination of IUD, balloon, estrogen, and hyaluronic acid reported a pregnancy rate of 314/475 (66%) with 201/314 (61%) resulting in a live birth[102]. A national referral center in the Netherlands reported menstrual outcomes for 638 consecutively treated women over a 10-year period[68]. The success rate, defined as normal menstruation, was 95%. However, recurrence of IUAs requiring up to three surgical interventions was reported in 27% of women; those with more severe adhesions at baseline were more likely to have a need for subsequent adhesiolysis.

The etiology for the development of IUAs also appears to impact outcome. Women with IUAs associated with uterine artery embolization[103] or uterine compression sutures placed for postpartum hemorrhage appear to have less favorable outcomes than those with adhesions secondary to intrauterine surgical trauma[104, 105]. The use of gel barriers has been the subject of a metaanalysis that notes that fertility outcomes are generally of poor quality[106]. A primary issue is that the RCTs examining this intervention report primarily on reduction of adhesion reformation and not on subsequent pregnancy. These pooled data do not suggest a benefit for any fertility outcome at this time, and it is essential that future studies report these data.

Recommendations for future research

Since the previous guidelines, there have been an increasing number of RCTs, particularly evaluating methods for primary and secondary prevention. Specific surgical techniques remain untested by RCTs; however, it is recognized that it would be difficult to investigate this aspect of treating IUAs, with surgical variation, protocol development, and adherence and recruitment issues being problematic. Specific future research pathways may include:

1. Methods of diagnosis that may be predictive of outcome. Sonography incorporating contrast agents, 3D reconstruction, Doppler or power flow studies, and MRI techniques may present new pathways for prognosis of treatment and

value when counseling women considering treatment.

2. Demonstrating fertility outcomes from RCTs examining primary and secondary prevention techniques. These are of particular importance given the most common presenting problem of IUAs is subfertility.

3. Further study of BMDSC treatment as a medical alternative to surgery, based on initial studies.

It is recognized that a universal classification system would benefit future research studies, although given the current limitations of any single classification system, this is unlikely to occur in the foreseeable future.

Appendix

This report was developed under the direction of the Practice Committee of the AAGL as a service to its members and other practicing clinicians. The members of the Practice Committee have reported the following financial interest or affiliation with corporations: Jason A. Abbott, FRANZCOG Ph. D. —Consultant: Hologic, Inc. , Stryker Endoscopy, Vifor Pharmaceuticals; Malcolm G. Munro, M. D. —Consultant: Aegea Medical, Boston Scientific Corp. , Inc. , Gynesonics, Hologic, Stock Ownership: Channel Medical; Sony S. Singh, M. D. , FRCSC, FACOG—Speakers Bureau: AbbVie, Allergan, Bayer Healthcare Corp. ; Stacey Scheib, M. D. —nothing to disclose; Tiffany R. Jackson, M. D. —nothing to disclose; Frank Jansen, M. D. , Ph. D. —nothing to disclose; E. Britton Chahine, M. D. , FACOG—nothing to disclose.

The members of the AAGL Guideline Development Committee for Intrauterine Adhesions reported financial interest or affiliation with corporations: Jason A. Abbott (Chair), FRANZCOG Ph. D—Consultant: Hologic, Inc. , Stryker Endoscopy, Vifor Pharmaceuticals; Malcolm G. Munro, M. D. —Consultant: Aegea Medical, Boston Scientific Corp. , Inc. , Gynesonics, Hologic, Stock Ownership: Channel Medical; Rebecca Deans, M. D. (nothing to disclose), Mark Hans Emanuel, M. D. —Stock ownership: Smith & Nephew Endoscopy, IQ Medical Ventures; from the European Society of Gynaecological Endoscopy

(EGSE): Attilio Di Spiezio Sardo, M. D., Ph. D. (nothing to disclose), Rudi Campo, M. D., Consultant: Karl Storz Endoscopy, Tutlingen, Germany; and Rudy Leon De Wilde, M. D., Ph. D. (Consultant: Nordic Pharma, Karl Storz, Gynesonics).

Competing interests

The authors declare that they have no competing interests other than the ones mentioned in the Appendix.

Consent for publication

Not applicable.

Ethics approval and consent to participate

Not applicable.

Publisher's Note

Springer Nature remains neutral with regard to jurisdictional claims in published maps and institutional affiliations.

Received: 30 January 2017 Accepted: 23 March 2017

附录 C 2019 加拿大子宫内膜增生指南

加拿大妇产科医学会的政策是在指南出版 5 年后对其内容进行审查，届时可对文件进行重新确认或修订，以反映实践中出现的新证据和变化。

第 392 号，2019 年 12 月

第 392 号指南——子宫内膜增生的分型和管理

实践的变更

- 加拿大广泛采用 WHO 子宫内膜增生分型标准。
- 左炔诺孕酮宫内系统在子宫内膜增生治疗中的应用。
- 治疗子宫内膜增生需行子宫切除术时，首选微创手术方式。

核心要点

- 支持采取 WHO 子宫内膜增生分型标准。
- 应鼓励和支持子宫内膜增生患者积极纠正可逆的子宫内膜癌高危因素。
- 推荐 LNG-IUS 作为无不典型增生的首选治疗方案。
- 子宫内膜增生的手术治疗应首选腹腔镜下全子宫切除术。

摘要

目的：本指南的目的是帮助初级保健医生和妇科医生对疑似子宫内膜增生的妇女进行初步评估，建议所有医疗服务人员使用 2014 版 WHO 子宫内膜增生分型标准，并指导子宫内膜增生患者采取最佳治疗。

目标人群：表现为疑似或确诊的子宫内膜增生的成年女性（18 岁及以上）。

治疗方案：讨论有关无不典型子宫内膜增生和不典型子宫内膜增生女性可以选择的药物治疗以及手术治疗。

指南更新：证据将在出版 5 年后进行审查，以决定是否应更新指南的全部或部分内容。然而，如果在 5 年周期之前公布了重要的新证据，审查进程可能会加快，以便对一些建议进行更为迅速的更新。

总结：

1. 除了与雌激素暴露相关的流行病学高危因素外，经间期出血和绝经后出血与子宫内膜增生的风险增加有关。应根据公布的算法进行子宫内膜取样，特别注意 40 岁或以上或体重指数为 30 kg/m² 或以上的妇女（中级证据）。

2. 大多数无不典型增生可通过药物治疗逆转，子宫切除术并非一线治疗，仅适用于某些特定情况（中级证据）。

3. 子宫内膜增生应首选腹腔镜全子宫切除术，与开腹手术相比，可减少围手术期的并发症和死亡率（高级证据）。

4. 如果无不典型子宫内膜增生患者采用子宫切除术，手术特征那么绝经后妇女也应该进行双侧输卵管卵巢切除术。由于良性疾病的年轻女性卵巢切除相关的死亡率和发病率增加，只建议绝经前妇女进行双侧输卵管卵巢切除术（中级证据）。

5. 不典型增生（AH）有恶变或进展为内膜癌的风险，首选子宫全切除术加双侧输卵管卵巢切除术。需考虑绝经前妇女的卵巢潴留（低级证据）。

6. 无证据支持对子宫内膜增生病例常规行冰冻病理检查（低级证据）。

7. 无证据支持 AH 患者常规行淋巴结切除（中级证据）。

8. 无足够证据支持子宫内膜切除术是无不典型增生的一线手术治疗方式（低级证据）。

9. 子宫内膜息肉合并子宫内膜增生的患者，应根据内膜增生的组织学分型进行相应治疗（低级证据）。

推荐：

1. 2019 年 SOCG 指南推荐采用 2014 版 WHO 子宫内膜增生分型标准（强推荐，低级证据）。对于疑似子宫内膜癌的患者，Pipelle 活检术是适用于门诊初步诊断的子宫内膜活检方法（强推荐，高级证据）。

2. 经过初始的观察随访或药物治疗后，仍反复出现 AUB 症状者，推荐再次行子宫内膜活检评估（强推荐，高级证据）。

3. 医生应评估子宫内膜增生患者有哪些可逆的高危因素，并对其进行医学宣教，帮助患者治疗或逆转此类高危因素（强推荐，高级证据）。

4. 无不典型增生患者可观察随访。若观察期间未达自行缓解或有异常子宫出血，可考虑药物治疗（弱推荐，低级证据）。

5. 推荐 LNG-IUS 为无不典型增生的一线治疗，其不良反应更少，内膜逆转后继续放置至 5 年（强推荐，中级证据）。

6. 口服/注射低剂量孕激素是可选的替代治疗（强推荐，高级证据）。推荐低剂量孕激素治疗至少 6 个月。内膜评估可在治疗期间或停药 3 周后进行，以确保采取正确的选择（强推荐，低级证据）。

7. 无不典型增生的手术指征（强推荐，高级证据）包括：患者无保留生育意愿，随访过程中进展为不典型增生或子宫内膜癌，治疗 12 个月内膜仍无逆转，完成孕激素规范治疗后复发，AUB 症状持续存在，拒绝进行随访或药物治疗。

8. 如有手术指征，推荐手术方式为全子宫＋双侧输卵管切除术，是否行双侧卵巢切除取决于绝经状态（强推荐，中级证据）。

9. 绝经前与绝经后 AH 患者均推荐全子宫＋双侧附件切除（强推荐，中级证据）。绝经前女性是否保留卵巢应个体化评估（强推荐，中级证据）。

10. 所有子宫内膜增生病例应避免行次全子宫切除术及子宫粉碎性切除术（强推荐，低级证据）。

引言

子宫内膜增生的发病率随着年龄的增长而增加，总体估计为每年每 10 万妇女中有 133 例。它在 30 岁以下的女性中很少出现，在 50~54 岁的女性中达到高峰[1]。遗传学的发展使人们对其发病机制有了新的认识，并改变了传统的 4 层分型标准，即单纯型与复杂型的不典型增生和无不典型增生。2014 年，世界卫生组织修改了 1994 年的分类，仅包括两类：无不典型增生和不典型增生，不典型增生或子宫内膜上皮内瘤变（EIN）[2,3]。不典型子宫内膜增生和无不典型子宫内膜增生的高危因素与子宫内膜样子宫内膜癌相同，可导致子宫内膜的内源性或外源性雌激素的非拮抗性暴露[4]。不典型子宫内膜增生被认为是 I 型子宫内膜癌的先兆病变，因为两者具有相似的基因改变和单克隆生长[4,5]。事实上，高达 60％的子宫内膜上皮内瘤变患者已经或将进展为浸润型子宫内膜癌[6]。无不典型增生很少发展为子宫内膜癌（1％~3％），两者的基因突变并不相同[2,7]。不典型增生患者需要更明确的治疗方法，而无不典型增生患者可以采取保守治疗。证据质量的评定采用评估、制定和评价分级建议（GRADE）方法框架中所述的标准（附表 C-1）。强推荐和弱推荐的解释见附表 C-2。

临床表现

高危因素：子宫内膜增生的高危因素可分为 3 种。①月经异常因素（如高龄或绝经后出血、未育或不孕、初潮早或绝经晚、排卵障碍、绝经过渡期和/或多囊卵巢综合征）；②医源性因素（如无孕激素拮抗的雌激素长期应用史或他莫昔芬长期治疗患者）；③并发症（肥胖、糖尿病、高血压或林奇综合征等）[8]。

症状：绝经前妇女的症状包括异常子宫出血（如规律、频率、持续时间紊乱和月经过多）以及经间期出血[9]。针对绝经前妇女的系统回顾中，与月经过多（0.11％，95％置信区间 0.04％~0.32％）相比，经间出血的子宫内膜癌风险更高（0.52％，95％置信区间 0.23％~1.16％）[10]。应研究任何绝经后出血情况。

查体结果：查体结果可以正常，也可以包括体重指数（BMI）升高和多囊卵巢综合征特征。应进行双侧子宫检查，如有必要，应进行诊断性宫腔镜检查和子宫内膜活检。子宫内膜取样应按照加拿大妇产科学会发布的指南[11,12]进行，针对40 岁或以上妇女、未接受药物治疗的妇女和年轻妇女的异常出血，根据其高危因素进行。

附表 C-1　GRADE 证据质量分级

推荐强度	定义
强推荐	干预措施利大于弊或弊大于利。
弱推荐[a]	当利弊不确定或无论质量高低的证据均显示利弊相当。
证据质量等级	**定义**
高｜++++	我们非常确信真实的效应值接近效应估计值。
中｜+++0	对效应估计值我们有中等程度的信心：真实值有可能接近估计值，但仍存在二者大不相同的可能性。
低｜++00	我们对效应估计值的确信程度有限。真实值可能与估计值大不相同。
极低｜+000	我们对效应估计值几乎没有信心：真实值很可能与估计值大不相同。

[a] 不应将弱推荐解读为低级证据或不确定性推荐。

GRADE 工作组，SCHÜNEMANN H，BROŻEK J，et al. GRADE 手册．GRADE 工作组，2013．

参见：http：//gdt. guidelinedevelopment. org/app/handbook/handbook. html．2019 年 4 月 15 日查阅。

附表 C-2　对强推荐和弱推荐的评判和解释

评判和解释	强推荐 "我们推荐"	弱推荐 "我们建议"
指导小组的评判	小组很清楚一种方案的有利结果超过了替代方案的结果。	小组不太清楚一种方案的有利结果是否超过了替代方案。
对患者的启示	在这种情况下，大多数人希望采取推荐的行动方案，只有一小部分人不愿意。	在这种情况下，大多数人会想要建议的行动方案，但许多人不会。
对临床医生的启示	大多数人应该接受干预。根据指南，采取这一推荐方案可作为质量标准或性能指标。	临床医生应该认识到，每个人都有不同选择，临床医生必须帮助每个人做出符合其价值观和偏好的管理决策。
对决策者的影响	在大多数情况下，该建议可作为政策采纳。	决策将需要各利益相关方进行大量讨论和积极参与。

年龄阈值的依据是，年龄较大 AUB 女性（≥45 岁）患 EH，其子宫内膜增生和子宫内膜癌的风险较年轻 AUB 高［子宫内膜增生，比值比（OR）3.85；95%CI 1.75～8.49，$P=0.01$，子宫内膜癌，OR 4.03；95%CI 1.54～10.5，$P=0.04$］[13]。在所有女性中，一个重要的高危因素是 BMI：1 项针对绝经前妇女的研究发现，与正常 BMI 相比，BMI≥30 kg/m^2 的 AUB 女性进展为不典型增生或内膜癌风险是 BMI 正常 AUB 女性的 4 倍（95%CI：1.36～11.74）[14]。对于绝经后出血，建议进行子宫内膜取样。

参见第 1 条总结。

子宫内膜增生的诊断工具和监测：任何子宫内膜增生或子宫内膜癌的疑似患者都应进行子宫内膜组织取样检查。有许多设备可用于进行子宫内膜活检，其中包括 Pipelle、Explora、Accurette 和 Novak。

子宫内膜取样方法：有强有力的证据表明，上述任何一种方法都能提供诊断子宫内膜增生所需的可靠性、有效性和耐受性。然而，2000 年，Dijkhuizen 等人[15]的荟萃分析（包括 39 项研究和 7 914 名患者）表明，Pipelle 活检术对诊断子宫内膜增生或子宫内膜癌最敏感。Pipelle 活检术对绝经前和绝经后妇女子宫内膜癌的诊断敏感性分别为 91% 和 99.6%，一项 Meta 显示，Pipelle 活检术对绝经前和绝经后子宫内膜癌的诊断敏感度分别为 91% 和 99.6%，对不典型增生的诊断敏感度分别为 81%。

这些方法被认为是"盲检"，它们通常对不到 50% 的子宫内膜腔进行取样。在某些情况下，它们可能无法提供足够数量的组织，因而不能进行正确诊断。诊断性宫腔镜取样活检适用于以下情况：内膜活检阴性，但临床高度可疑子宫内膜增生或子宫内膜癌，持续性阴道流血，宫颈狭窄、子宫内膜活检失败，子宫内膜取样中取材不满意，过度疼痛/焦虑的患者。诊断性宫腔镜检查与直接取样和刮宫是这些情况的首选研究方法。

参见第 1 和第 2 条推荐。

宫腔镜检查或生理盐水灌注导致肿瘤外溢的风险：以前用宫腔镜或生理盐水超声检查子宫内膜增生或子宫内膜癌的妇女中，曾有肿瘤溢出和癌症恶化的担忧。自 2014 年以来，腹膜冲洗已不再是国际妇产科联合会子宫内膜癌分期的一部分。目前尚无前瞻性或回顾性研究显示，接受过内镜诊断程序的患者有任何不良后果。

组织病理学注意事项

世界卫生组织采用子宫内膜增生的二级或二元分型标准，以提高观察者间的可重复性（附表 C-3）：无不典型增生与不典型增生的比较[16]。

附表 C-3 2014 版 WHO 子宫内膜增生分型标准

2014 WHO 分型	包含术语	遗传谱	合并浸润型子宫内膜癌风险	进展为侵袭性子宫内膜癌的风险
无不典型子宫内膜增生	良性子宫内膜增生 单纯性不典型子宫内膜增生 复杂性不典型子宫内膜增生 单纯性无不典型子宫内膜增生 复杂性无不典型子宫内膜增生	低水平的体细胞突变	<1%	RR 1.01~1.03

2014 WHO 分型	包含术语	遗传谱	合并浸润型子宫内膜癌风险	进展为侵袭性子宫内膜癌的风险
不典型增生	复杂性不典型子宫内膜增生 单纯性不典型子宫内膜增生 子宫内膜上皮内瘤变（EIN）	微卫星不稳定性 *PAX2*、失活 *PTEN*、*KRAS* 和 *CTNNB1*（b-catenin）突变	高达60%	RR 14~45

注：*CTNNB1*：连环蛋白 β1；*KRAS*：v-Ki-ras2 Kirsten 大鼠肉瘤病毒癌基因同源物；*PAX2*：配对 box 基因 2；*PTEN*：磷酸酶和张力蛋白类似物。

来自 Abu Hashim 等人[2]和 Emons 等人的数据[3]。

无不典型增生的组织病理：子宫内膜可能表现息肉样和囊性增厚，但也可能是可变的。显微镜下，腺体大小和形状各异，腺上皮内呈不规则的囊性轮廓和有丝分裂样结构，而间质数量是多变的。良性子宫内膜息肉，尤其是呈碎片状时，腺体可能不规则/扩张，可被误解为无不典型增生；然而，虽然息肉是局灶性的，但无不典型增生是弥散性的。另一个发现是"增生性子宫内膜紊乱"，即腺体的不规则性超过正常的增生性子宫内膜，但未出现无不典型增生。

不典型增生（子宫内膜上皮内瘤变）的组织病理学：子宫内膜也可能增厚和息肉样，但这是可变的。显微镜下，复杂的腺体密集（导致间质减少），伴有核异型性（>1 mm），这与相邻的未受累腺体明显不同。良性化生样和假性腺体样病变应排除在外。镜下不典型增生缺乏子宫内膜样腺癌的间质增生和广泛的腺体融合。

孕激素治疗增生的组织病理学：孕激素治疗可改变增生的外观（例如，假性蜕膜化可减轻腺体拥挤和细胞学上的不典型性）[17]。因此，接受孕激素治疗时，当再次活检没有增生不应被解释为清除。另一方面，孕激素治疗后的残留病灶被标记为"孕激素治疗的非典型增生"[17]。

在孕激素治疗结束后，一些权威机构建议每6个月重新活检一次，出院前连续两次活检阴性，尽管根据高危因素和异常出血的复发情况，监测可能会增加。

管理

处理高危因素：医生应告知患者肥胖与子宫内膜增生/内膜癌有密切关系，并鼓励患者减肥[18,19]。事实上，子宫内膜增生患者治疗目标的一部分就是纠正这些医疗状况[20]。

参见第 3 条推荐。

无不典型子宫内膜增生：

初期管理：相对良性的自然病史支持了无不典型内膜增生的保育治疗的初步尝试。随访长达 20 年的队列研究评估了进展为子宫内膜癌的长期风险小于 5%[21-23]。此外，据报道，在选择等待观察的患者中，自发消退率为 75%～100%[21,22]。

参见第 4 条推荐。

治疗方案选择：有大量文献支持口服孕激素和左炔诺孕酮宫内节育系统（LNG-IUS）治疗绝经前和绝经后无不典型子宫内膜增生患者的有效性。口服孕激素组和 LNG-IUS 组无不典型子宫内膜增生的疾病消退率分别为 67%～72% 和 81%～94%，在最近的 2 项荟萃分析中，包括总共 8 项随机对照试验[24-31]。注射用醋酸甲羟孕酮也可被视为 LNG-IUS 的替代方案，6 个月时消退率达到 92%[32]。LNG-IUS 的有效性和较小的副作用使其成为无不典型子宫内膜增生患者的首选治疗方法。芳香化酶抑制剂也是无不典型子宫内膜增生患者的有效治疗选择。最近进行的一项随机对照试验[33]发现，来曲唑的疗效与醋酸甲地孕酮相当，并且副作用较少，可用于绝经前和绝经后妇女。附表 C-4 概述了孕激素在子宫内膜增生保育治疗中的应用。

治疗时间和随访：为诱导子宫内膜增生的消退，而不出现非典型性症状，通常必须至少维持 6 个月的口服孕激素或 LNG-IUS 治疗[34]。应该通过子宫内膜取样进行治疗反应的随访，这可以在宫内节育器在位的情况下进行。通常每 3～6 个月进行一次子宫内膜活检，以确保治疗期间没有疾病进展[5,20]。如药物治疗 6 个月仍未逆转，可根据个体情况决定是否继续当前治疗[35]。如药物治疗 12 个月仍未逆转，应考虑改用其他治疗方案[5]。

孕激素治疗通常持续 6 个月，而 LNG-IUS 在出现治疗反应的患者中维持 5 年[5,36]。已证实接受孕激素治疗的患者和体重指数为 35 kg/m² 或更高的患者复发率更高[37]。因此，这些患者的随访时间应延长[38]。

参见第 5 和第 6 条推荐。

手术治疗的适应证：对于不希望保留生育能力，以及在随访中发展为不典型增生或进展为癌的患者，药物治疗 12 个月后增生仍未消退或完成治疗后复发，尽管接受了治疗仍有持续异常子宫出血，或拒绝子宫内膜监测或药物治疗的患者，手术治疗应予以保留[39]。手术治疗将另行讨论。

参考第 7 条推荐。

不典型子宫内膜增生/子宫内膜上皮内瘤变：

初期管理：高达 60％的子宫内膜上皮内瘤变患者已经或将要发展为浸润性子宫内膜癌[7]，因此，全子宫切除联合双侧输卵管卵巢切除术（BSO）是该类病患的首选治疗方法。手术治疗另行讨论。

附表 C-4　孕激素在子宫内膜增生保留生育能力治疗中的应用

孕激素	用法及剂量		商品名	常用剂量
MPA	连续口服	大剂量	Provera	$100\sim200$ mg/d
		低剂量		$2.5\sim20$ mg/d
	口服周期			$10\sim20$ mg/d×$10\sim12$ d/周期
	注射		Depo-Provera	每 90 天 150 mg
MA	大剂量		Megace	$80\sim320$ mg/d
	低剂量			40 mg/d
NETA	连续口服		Norlutate	$5\sim15$ mg/d
	口服周期			15 mg/d×$10\sim12$ d/周期
孕激素			Prometrium	$100\sim300$ mg/d
LNG-IUS			Mirena	20 μg/d

注：LNG-IUS：左炔诺孕酮宫内节育系统；MA：醋酸甲地孕酮；MPA：醋酸甲羟孕酮；NETA：炔诺酮。

治疗方案选择和随访：对于希望保留生育能力或医学上不适合手术的患者可考虑保留子宫。咨询很重要，不仅要考虑子宫内膜癌的潜在风险，还应包括子宫内膜癌高于Ⅰ期（2％）、并发卵巢癌（4％）和死亡（0.5％）的风险[40]。在非对照的系统评价中，这些结果很难通过治疗前的调查来预测[40]。保留生育能力的治疗目标包括完全逆转疾病、恢复子宫内膜的正常功能和预防侵袭性疾病；然而对于状况较差的手术候选人来说，医疗治疗的目标是稳定疾病和预防癌症[41]。

保育治疗方案包括孕激素（口服或局部）、芳香化酶抑制剂或促性腺激素释放激素激动剂。附表 C-4 显示了可用于治疗子宫内膜上皮内瘤变的孕激素类型和剂量。通常治疗 6 个月后评估内膜逆转情况，治疗 12 个月，大多数患者内膜实现逆转[40,42]。逆转率 55%～92%，复发率 3%～55%[33,40,42-45]。甚至在没有代谢综合征的情况下，二甲双胍也可以增加治疗效果[46,47]。值得注意的是，肥胖可能会降低逆转率[43]。每 3 个月进行 1 次子宫内膜评估，直至连续 2 次内膜活检阴性[34,40]。治疗结束后 2 年内复发风险最高，建议每 6 个月行 1 次内膜评估，持续 2 年。此后每年进行 1 次，直至去除危险因素或手术治疗[37,48]。随访过程中进展为子宫内膜癌，治疗 12 个月内膜仍无逆转，或完成孕激素规范治疗后复发，AUB 症状持续存在，或者拒绝进行随访或药物治疗的患者应接受明确的手术治疗[39]。如患者不适合手术，复发后可进行第 2 轮孕激素治疗，预期逆转率 85%。如二次复发，可进行第 3 轮孕激素治疗[49]。

　　子宫内膜上皮内瘤变保留生育能力治疗：子宫内膜上皮内瘤变患者如果希望保留生育能力，应尽早咨询生殖内分泌科医生，因为他们有疾病复发和生育能力低下的风险[40]。保留生育能力的选择包括在子宫联合 BSO 术前进行卵母细胞或胚胎冷冻保存，随后进行辅助生殖技术治疗，以及保留卵巢的子宫切除术和未来待孕的方式[50,55]。医疗服务人员应将这些患者转诊给妇科肿瘤医生，因为潜在的肿瘤相当常见[51]。应鼓励女性保持体重指数在 30 kg/m^2 以下，因为复发在肥胖患者中更为常见[51,52]。比较进行初始子宫切除术和为保留生育力而延迟进行子宫切除术的患者时发现，癌症发病率似乎并未增加[53]。事实上，不孕治疗似乎不会增加 EIN 的复发率[54]。经保留生育能力治疗后的活产率为 7%～26%，妊娠与疾病复发的概率较低有关[34,40,42,54]。当疾病复发的风险较高，且不再需要生育时，建议行子宫 BSO 切除术[41,56]。

外科治疗

　　无不典型子宫内膜增生症的手术适应证：全子宫切除术为无非典型性子宫内膜增生症提供了明确的治疗方法，但这也是一个与并发症和生育能力丧失相关的手术方式。一般来说，子宫切除术适用于，如尽管使用孕激素仍有持久性或复发性增生，进展为不典型增生或癌，持续存在的异常子宫出血和患者的偏好选择。手术也同样适用于对药物治疗不耐受或有禁忌证、不能或不愿意接受持续监测、未来没有生育需求以及子宫内膜癌高基线风险的患者[36,56]。

无不典型子宫内膜增生症的手术治疗应包括全子宫切除术＋卵管切除术＋切除双侧卵巢或不切除双侧卵巢[39]。绝经后妇女卵巢通常被切除。然而，在绝经前患者尤其是 45 岁以下的患者中，由于年轻女性存在与双侧卵巢切除术相关的全因死亡率和发病率的长期风险，应考虑保留卵巢[57]。在子宫切除时仅行预防性输卵管切除术，可降低原位保留卵巢时的卵巢癌风险[58]。

参见第 2 条总结。

不典型子宫内膜增生/子宫内膜上皮内瘤变：全子宫切除联合 BSO 术是不典型子宫内膜增生症的首选治疗方法，因为其进展为恶性肿瘤或并发子宫内膜癌的风险很高[23,59]。

观察性研究表明，高达 60% 报告为无典型子宫内膜增生的子宫内膜活检标本中发现了潜在的癌细胞[59-64]。出于同样的原因，一般建议绝经前和绝经后妇女在全子宫切除的基础上进行 BSO 术。应充分讨论绝经前患有良性疾病的妇女因双侧卵巢切除术而导致死亡率和发病率增加的风险，并针对每个个体制订治疗方案[56]。

手术入路：目前尚无证据指导无不典型子宫内膜增生的子宫切除术的手术入路选择。考虑到这种病理亚型被认为是一种非肿瘤性实体[64]，阴道、腹腔镜和开放手术都均是可以接受的。无论是经阴道或腹腔镜行良性病变子宫切除术，其围手术期并发症较少[6]。

不典型子宫内膜增生与潜在患癌的高风险相关，因此，手术路径应包括对其附件和其他盆腔结构是否有侵袭性疾病的迹象进行评估。与开放手术相比，腹腔镜手术可减少围手术期并发症，缩短住院时间，并能更快恢复正常活动[65]。即使是子宫内膜癌，腹腔镜手术与开腹手术相比，生存结果相似[65]。因此，对于不典型子宫内膜增生，应首先考虑微创子宫切除术，而子宫切除术仅限于不可行的病例。

由于担心恶性肿瘤和肿瘤弥散，所有子宫内膜增生的病例应避免行子宫次全切除术和子宫壁剥离术[39]。

参见第 3、第 4 和第 5 条总结。

参见第 8、第 9 和第 10 条总结。

其他手术注意事项：关于因对子宫内膜增生病例行冰冻病理检查以排除癌症的相关文献的结论是不一致的，并且仅限于小规模的观察性研究[66-72]。有几篇报告赞成在术中进行冷冻切片以确定哪些患者需要进行癌症分期手术[68-72]。

这种方法的一个局限性是冰冻病理检查和最终病理结果可能不一致，这可能导致在手术中出现过度治疗或治疗不足[67]。此外，中心机构可能没有内部的病理学家进行冰冻病理检查，且如有必要，也可能没有熟练的专业医生进行淋巴结切除术。如果子宫切除术后的最终病理诊断为子宫内膜癌，通常分化良好，并且与需要额外手术分期的高风险特征无关[59,66,73]。在没有冰冻病理检查的中心机构进行子宫内膜增生手术是合理的[66]。因为总体来说，无足够的证据支持在子宫内膜增生病例常规行冰冻病理检查。

参见第 6 条总结。

目测：外科医生对子宫的大体检查是另一种评估子宫肌层浸润深度和术中盆腔淋巴结切除必要性的方法。但支持这一做法的可用数据很少[74,75]。然而，我们应该意识到，对标本不准确的视觉评价可能导致错误的手术决定。因为它可能损坏标本，从而干扰正确的病理分析，因而这种做法是不提倡的。

淋巴结切除术：尽管不典型子宫内膜增生患者存在潜在的恶性肿瘤风险，但包括盆腔淋巴结切除术在内的手术分期将导致大多数患者过度治疗[59,76]。由于高风险癌变的发生率较低，且考虑到子宫切除时行淋巴结切除会增加手术风险，因此最初更倾向于保留生育能力治疗[59,76]。2015 年的一项 Cochrane 综述显示，没有证据支持早期子宫内膜癌常规淋巴结切除术[76]；然而，随着前哨淋巴结评估成为常规做法并取代了完整的淋巴结切除，各个中心的做法也各不相同。冰冻病理检查或最终病理诊断为子宫内膜癌的所有病例，均应咨询妇科肿瘤科，以确定治疗方法。

参见第 7 条总结。

子宫内膜去除术：有报道称，子宫内膜切除术和消融术可成功地长期治疗无不典型子宫内膜增生[64,77]。最大的前瞻性研究，包括 161 例因单纯性无不典型子宫内膜增生和复杂性无不典型增生而行子宫内膜切除或消融术的患者[64]。其中位随访时间为 7 年，大多数患者（95.7%）没有出现进一步出血或疼痛症状。12 名患者在随访期间进行了子宫内膜切除术，最终病理结果没有发现任何持续性增生[64]。作者确定子宫内膜消融术是治疗无不典型子宫内膜增生的一种安全的方法[64]。但这种技术的一个局限性是难以确定子宫内膜是否被完全破坏。由于子宫内膜腔的闭塞，持续监测也具有挑战性，这是子宫内膜癌持续高危因素患者特别关注的原因。

目前没有足够的证据支持子宫内膜切除术作为无不典型子宫内膜增生的一线治疗方法，除非在禁止大手术的情况下。如果是在子宫内膜消融术完成后偶然获得诊断的情况下，则无须进一步治疗，尤其是子宫内膜切除术[64]。应定期对患者进行随访，并检查异常出血是否持续或复发。

不典型增生是一种癌前状态，因此不典型子宫内膜增生患者通常避免行子宫内膜切除术或消融术。在这些情况下，子宫内膜切除术或消融术不建议用于不适合进行相关手术的患者，应与妇科肿瘤医生充分商讨后再做决定。

参见第 8 条总结。

子宫内膜息肉中子宫内膜增生的治疗：当子宫内膜息肉内诊断为子宫内膜增生时，即使宫腔镜下内膜影像正常，仍建议对 EP 周围的内膜组织取样。约 52%的病例发现 EP 周围内膜存在无不典型/不典型增生[78]。对 10 项主要是回顾性研究的系统评价显示，子宫内膜息肉伴不典型增生患者有 5.6%合并有子宫内膜癌[79]。子宫内膜息肉合并子宫内膜增生的患者，应根据内膜增生的组织学分型进行相应治疗。

参见第 9 条总结。

［注］参考文献见英文版。

李雪英　吴岭

Guideline No. 392－Classification and Management of Endometrial Hyperplasia

KEY MESSAGES

• A universal system for classification that follows the World Health Organization classification for endometrial hyperplasia should be used.

• Patients should receive encouragement and support to modify reversible risk factors for endometrial cancer.

• The levonorgestrel intrauterine system should be used as the first-line treatment for endometrial hyperplasia without atypia.

• A minimally invasive approach hysterectomy is preferred for endometrial hyperplasia.

Abstract

Objective: The aim of this guideline is to aid primary care physicians and gynaecologists in the initial evaluation of women with suspected endometrial hyperplasia, to recommend the use of the 2014 World Health Organization classification for endometrial hyperplasia by all health care providers, and to guide the optimal treatment of women diagnosed with endometrial hyperplasia.

Intended Users: Physicians, including gynaecologists, obstetricians, family physicians, general surgeons, emergency medicine specialists; nurses, including registered nurses and nurse practitioners; medical trainees, including medical students, residents, and fellows; and all other health care providers.

Target Population: Adult women (18 years and older) presenting with suspected or confirmed endometrial hyperplasia.

Options: The discussion relates to the medical therapy as well as surgical treatment options for women with and without atypical endometrial hyperplasia.

Evidence: For this guideline, relevant studies were searched in PubMed, CochraneWiley, and the Cochrane Systematic Reviews using the following terms, either alone or in combination, with the search limited to English language materials, human subjects, and published since 2000: (endometrial hyperplasia, endometrial intraepithelial neoplasia, endometrial sampling, endometrial curettage, diagnosis) AND (treatment, progestin therapy, surgery, LNG-IUS, aromatase inhibitors, metformin), AND (obesity). The search was performed in April 2018. Relevant evidence was selected for inclusion in the following order: meta-analyses, systematic reviews, guidelines, randomized controlled trials, prospective cohort studies, observational studies, non-systematic reviews, case series, and reports. Additional significant articles were identified through cross-referencing the identified reviews. The total number of studies identified was 2152, and 82 studies were included in this review.

Validation Methods: The content and recommendations were drafted and a-greed upon by the authors. The Executive and Board of the Society of Gynecologic Oncology of Canada reviewed the content and submitted comments for consideration, and the Board of the Society of Obstetricians and Gynaecologists of Canada approved the final draft for publication. The quality of evidence was rated using the criteria described in the Grading of Recommendations Assessment, Development and Evaluation (GRADE) methodology framework. The interpretation of strong and weak recommendations was also included. The Summary of Findings is available upon request.

Benefits, Harms, and/or Costs: It is expected that this guideline will benefit women with endometrial hyperplasia. This should guide patient informed consent before both medical and surgical management of this condition.

Guideline Update: Evidence will be reviewed 5 years after publication to decide whether all or part of the guideline should be updated. However, if important new evidence is published prior to the 5-year cycle, the review process may be accelerated for a more rapid update of some recommendations.

Summary Statements:

1. In addition to epidemiologic risk factors related to estrogen exposure, intermenstrual bleeding and postmenopausal bleeding are associated with increased risk of endometrial hyperplasia. Endometrial sampling should be carried out as per published algorithms with particular attention to women 40 years or older or with a body mass index of 30 kg/m^2 or greater (moderate).

2. Since the majority of cases of endometrial hyperplasia without atypia are successfully managed medically, hysterectomy is not considered first-line treatment and surgery is reserved for specific circumstances (moderate).

3. A minimally invasive approach to hysterectomy is preferred for endometrial hyperplasia as it decreases perioperative morbidity and mortality (high).

4. If hysterectomy is indicated for endometrial hyperplasia without atypia then postmenopausal women should also be offered bilateral salpingo-oophorectomy. This decision is individualized for premenopausal women due to increased

mortality and morbidity associated with removal of the ovaries in young women with benign disease (moderate).

5. Hysterectomy and bilateral salpingo-oophorectomy are the recommended treatment for atypical endometrial hyperplasia due to the underlying risk of malignancy or progression to endometrial cancer. Retention of the ovaries in premenopausal women may be considered (low).

6. There is no evidence to support routine intraoperative frozen section analysis in cases of endometrial hyperplasia (low).

7. There is no evidence to support routine lymphadenectomy for atypical endometrial hyperplasia (moderate).

8. There is insufficient evidence to support endometrial ablation as first-line surgical treatment for endometrial hyperplasia without atypia (low).

9. Endometrial hyperplasia found in endometrial polyps should be treated according to its histologic classification (low).

Recommendations:

1. Health care providers should use the 2014 World Health Organization histopathologic classification of endometrial hyperplasia (strong, low). If endometrial cancer is suspected, endometrial tissue sampling using a Pipelle device in an outpatient setting is the most appropriate first step for diagnosis (strong, high).

2. Those with recurrent symptoms of abnormal uterine bleeding after initial observation or medical treatment should be reassessed with an endometrial biopsy (strong, high).

3. Patients with endometrial hyperplasia should be assessed for reversible risk factors and receive education and support from their clinicians in order to treat and reverse those conditions (strong, high).

4. Patients with endometrial hyperplasia without atypia can be observed. They can be offered hormonal treatment if hyperplasia does not resolve with observation or experience abnormal uterine bleeding (weak, low).

5. The levonorgestrel intrauterine system should be used as the first-line treatment for endometrial hyperplasia without atypia due to its effectiveness and

favourable side effect profile (strong, high) and due to the fact that it can be kept in place for 5 years in patients showing treatment response (strong, moderate).

6. Low-dose oral and injectable progestins remain an acceptable treatment option for women with endometrial hyperplasia with and without atypia desiring an alternative treatment modality (strong, high). For patients on oral progestins, we suggest starting on a low dose for a minimum of 6 months. We suggest that assessment of the endometrium be done mid-therapy as well as 3 weeks after completion of treatment to ensure proper interpretation (strong, very low).

7. Surgical treatment of endometrial hyperplasia without atypia should be reserved for patients who do not want to preserve their fertility and experience progression to atypical hyperplasia or carcinoma during follow-up, whose hyperplasia fails to regress after 12 months of medical treatment or relapses after completing treatment with progestins, who continue to experience abnormal uterine bleeding despite treatment, or who decline endometrial surveillance or medical treatment (strong, high).

8. If surgery is indicated for endometrial hyperplasia without atypia, the procedure should include total hysterectomy with opportunistic salpingectomy, with or without bilateral oophorectomy depending on menopausal status (strong, moderate).

9. Total hysterectomy with bilateral salpingo-oophorectomy is recommended for treatment of atypical hyperplasia in premenopausal and postmenopausal women (strong, moderate). In premenopausal women, ovarian preservation should be discussed (strong, moderate).

10. We recommend that subtotal (supracervical) hysterectomy and morcellation be avoided in all cases of endometrial hyperplasia (strong, low).

INTRODUCTION

The incidence of endometrial hyperplasia increases with age, with an overall estimate of 133 per 100 000 woman-years. It is rarely seen in women under the age of 30 and reaches its peak in women aged 50 to 54. [1] Advances in genetics have led to a new understanding of its pathogenesis and a modification of the tra-ditional 4-tier classification of simple and complex hyperplasia with and without atypia. In 2014, the World Health Organization modified the 1994 classification to include only 2 categories: (1) hyperplasia without atypia and (2) hyperplasia with atypia: atypical hyperplasia or endometrial intraepithelial neoplasia (EIN). [2,3] The risk factors associated with endometrial hyperplasia with or with-out atypia are the same as those associated with endometrioid endometrial carcino-mas and result in unopposed estrogen exposure of the endometrium from endoge-nous or exogenous sources. [4] Atypical endometrial hyperplasia is thought to be a precursor lesion to type I endometrial carcinomas as both share a similar profile of genetic alterations and monoclonal growth. [4,5] In fact, up to 60% of patients with EIN have already developed or will develop an invasive endometrial cancer. [6] Hyperpla-sia without atypia rarely progresses to endometrial carcinoma (1%−3%), and it does not share the same genetic mutations as its counterpart. [2,7] Whereas atypical hy-perplasia warrants a more definitive treatment approach, non-atypical hyperplasia can be managed conservatively. The quality of evidence was rated using the crite-ria described in the Grading of Recommendations Assessment, Development and Evaluation (GRADE) methodology framework (Table 1). The interpretation of strong and weak recommendations is described in Table 2.

CLINICAL PRESENTATION

Risk Factors

Risk factors for endometrial hyperplasia can be divided into (1) menstrual factors (e. g. , older age or postmenopausal status, nulliparity or infertility, early menarche or later menopause, anovulation, menopausal transition and/or poly-cystic ovarian syndrome; (2) iatrogenic factors (e. g. , unopposed exogenous es-trogen therapy or tamoxifen); and (3) comorbidities (e. g. , obesity, diabetes, hypertension, or Lynch syndrome). [8]

Table 1. Key to Grading of Recommendations, Assessment, Development and Evaluation (GRADE)

Strength of the recommendation	Definition
Strong	Highly confident of the balance between desirable and undesirable consequences (i. e. , desirable consequences outweigh the undesirable consequences; or undesirable consequences outweigh the desirable consequences).
Conditional (weak)[a]	Less confident of the balance between desirable and undesirable consequences.
Quality level of a body of evidence	Definition
High++++	We are very confident that the true effect lies close to that of the estimate of the effect.
Moderate+++0	We are moderately confident in the effect estimate: The true effect is likely to be close to the estimate of the effect, but there is a possibility that it is substantially different.
Low++00	Our confidence in the effect estimate is limited. The true effect may be substantially different from the estimate of the effect.
Very low+000	We have very little confidence in the effect estimate: The true effect is likely to be substantially different from the estimate of effect

[a] Conditional (weak) recommendations should not be misinterpreted as weak evidence or uncertainty of the recommendation.

GRADE Working Group, Schünemann H, Broźek J, et al, (editors). The GRADE Handbook. GRADE Working Group; 2013. Available at: http: //gdt. guidelinedevelopment. org/app/handbook/handbook. html. Accessed on April 15, 2019.

Table 2. Judgement and interpretation of strong and conditional recommendations

Judgement/ Interpretation	Strong recommendation "We recommend..."	Conditional recommendation "We suggest..."
Judgement by guideline panel	It is clear to the panel that the net desirable consequences of a strategy outweighed the consequences of the alternative strategy.	It is less clear to the panel whether the net desirable consequences of a strategy outweighed the alternative strategy.
Implications for patients	Most individuals in this situation would want the recommended course of action, and only a small proportion would not.	Most individuals in this situation would want the suggested course of action, but many would not.
Implications for clinicians	Most individuals should receive the intervention. Adherence to this recommendation according to the guideline could be used as a quality criterion or performance indicator.	Clinicians should recognize that different choices will be appropriate for each individual and that clinicians must help each individual to arrive at a management decision consistent with his or her values and preferences.
Implications for policy makers	The recommendation can be adopted as policy in most situations.	Policy making will require substantial debate and involvement of various stakeholders.

Symptoms

In premenopausal women, symptoms include abnormal uterine bleeding (e. g., disturbances in regularity, frequency, duration, and heaviness of menstrual bleeding) as well as intermenstrual bleeding.[9] In a systematic review of premenopausal women, risk of endometrial carcinoma was higher with intermenstrual bleeding (0. 52%, 95% confidence interval [CI] 0. 23%−1. 16%) compared with heavy menstrual bleeding (0. 11%, 95% CI 0. 04%−0. 32%). [10] Any instances of postmenopausal bleeding should be investigated.

Physical Findings

Physical exam findings can be normal or include an elevated body mass index (BMI) and features of polycystic ovarian syndrome. Bimanual exam of the uterus should be performed, followed by a speculum exam for Pap testing if indicated and endometrial biopsy. Endometrial sampling should be performed following the Society of Obstetricians and Gynaecologists of Canada published guidelines[11,12] for abnormal bleeding in women age 40 or older, in those not responding to medical therapy, and in younger women based on their risk factors. The rationale for the age cut-off is that the risks of endometrial hyperplasia and carcinoma were significantly higher for abnormal bleeding in older women than in younger women (for age$\geqslant$45, odds ratio [OR] 3. 85; 95% CI 1. 75−8. 49, $P=0.01$, for hyperplasia, and OR 4. 03; 95% CI 1. 54−10. 5, $P=0.04$, for carcinoma). [13] In all women, an important risk factor is BMI: 1 study found that a BMI of 30 kg/m² or greater conveyed significantly higher risk of endometrial hyperplasia/carcinoma compared with normal BMI (OR 4. 00; 95% CI 1. 36−11. 74), controlling for age in premenopausal women. [14] For postmenopausal bleeding, endometrial sampling is recommended.

REFERS TO SUMMARY STATEMENT 1

Diagnostic Tools and Surveillance for Endometrial Hyperplasia

Any woman with suspected endometrial hyperplasia or endometrial cancer should be investigated with endometrial tissue sampling. Numerous devices are available for performing an endometrial biopsy; among them are the Pipelle, the Explora, the Accurette, and the Novak.

Endometrial sampling methods

There is strong evidence that any of the aforementioned methods offers the reliability, effectiveness, and tolerability required to diagnose endometrial hyperplasia. However, the meta-analysis from Dijkhuizen et al. [15] in 2000 that includes 39 studies and 7914 patients, showed that the Pipelle device was the most sensitive for diagnosing endometrial hyperplasia or endometrial cancer. The diagnostic sensitivity of the Pipelle device was 91% and 99.6% for detecting endometrial cancer in premenopausal and postmenopausal women, respectively and 81% for detecting atypical hyperplasia.

These methods are considered "blind approaches", and they usually sample less than 50% of the endometrial cavity. In certain circumstances they may fail to provide a sufficient amount of tissue and hence inhibit a proper diagnosis. In such a scenario, additional or alternative methods for endometrial sampling will be necessary. Any patient with either a non-diagnostic or benign endometrial sample with remaining high suspicion of endometrial hyperplasia or cancer, persistent bleeding, cervical stenosis, failed endometrial biopsy, or excessive pain/anxiety should be offered an additional or alternative diagnostic strategy. Diagnostic hysteroscopy with directed sampling and curettage is the preferred method of investigation in these situations.

REFERS TO RECOMMENDATIONS 1 & 2

Risk of Tumour Spillage Through Hysteroscopy or Saline Infusion

There were concerns about tumour spillage and cancer upstaging in women previously investigated with hysteroscopy or saline ultrasound for endometrial hyperplasia or cancer. Since 2014, peritoneal washing has not been part of the International Federation of Gynecology and Obstetrics staging for endometrial cancer. There is no prospective or retrospective study showing any adverse outcome for patients with a previous endoscopic diagnostic procedure.

HISTOPATHOLOGIC CONSIDERATIONS

The World Health Organization adopted a 2-tier or binary classification of endometrial hyperplasia in order to improve interobserver reproducibility (Table 3): hyperplasia without atypia versus hyperplasia with atypia. [16]

Table 3. 2014 World Health Organization classification of endometrial hyperplasia

2014 Terminology	Synonyms	Genetic profile	Coexistent invasive endometrial carcinoma	Risk of progression to invasive endometrial carcinoma
Hyperplasia without atypia	Benign endometrial hyperplasia Simple non-atypical endometrial hyperplasia Complex non-atypical endometrial hyperplasia Simple endometrial hyperplasia without atypia Complex endometrial hyperplasia without atypia	Low levels of somatic mutations	<1%	RR 1.01 −1.03
Hyperplasia with atypia	Complex atypical endometrial hyperplasia Simple atypical endometrial hyperplasia Endometrial intraepithelial neoplasia (EIN)	Microsatellite instability $PAX2$ inactivation $PTEN$, $KRAS$, and $CTNNB1$ (β-catenin) mutations	Up to 60%	RR 14−45

$CTNNB1$: catenin beta 1; $KRAS$: v-Ki-ras2 Kirsten rat sarcoma viral oncogene homologue; $PAX2$: paired box gene 2; $PTEN$: phosphatase and tensin analogue.

Data from Abu Hashim et al. [2] and Emons et al. [3]

Histopathology of Hyperplasia Without Atypia

The endometrium may appear thickened with polypoid and cystic areas but can be variable. Microscopically, glands vary in size and shape, with irregular and cystic outlines with mitotic figures in the glandular epithelium, while the amount of stroma is variable. Benign endometrial polyps, particularly when fragmented, can have irregular/dilated glands and be misinterpreted as hyperplasia without atypia; however, while polyps are focal, hyperplasia without atypia is diffuse. Another finding is "disordered proliferative endometrium", where glandular irregularity exceeds normal proliferative endometrium but falls short of hyperplasia without atypia.

Histopathology of Atypical Hyperplasia (Endometrial Intraepithelial Neoplasia)

The endometrium may also be thickened and polypoid, but this can be variable. Microscopically, complex glands are crowded (resulting in diminished stroma) with nuclear atypia (>1 mm in size), which is distinctly different from adjacent unaffected glands. Benign metaplastic and artifactual glandular mimics should be excluded. On microscopic examination, atypical hyperplasia lacks the stromal desmoplasia and extensive glandular confluence of endometrioid adenocarcinoma.

Histopathology of Progestin-Treated Hyperplasia

Progestin therapy can change the appearance of hyperplasia (e. g., pseudo-decidualization appears to lessen glandular crowding and cytologic atypia). [17] Thus, the absence of hyperplasia on a re-biopsy while on progestin therapy should not be interpreted as clearance. On the other hand, residual disease while on progestin therapy is labelled "progestin-treated atypical hyperplasia". [17] After the completion of progestin therapy, some authorities recommend rebiopsy every 6 months, with 2 consecutive negative biopsies prior to discharge, although surveillance may increase depending on risk factors and recurrence of abnormal bleeding.

MANAGEMENT

Addressing the Risk Factors

Physicians have an important role to play in educating patients about the relationship between obesity and endometrial hyperplasia/cancer and encouraging them to lose weight. [18,19] In fact, part of the therapeutic goals for patients with endometrial hyperplasia is the correction of those medical conditions. [20]

REFERS TO RECOMMENDATION 3

Endometrial Hyperplasia Without Atypia

Initial management

An initial attempt at conservative management of endometrial hyperplasia without atypia is supported by its relatively benign natural history. Cohort studies with up to 20 years of follow-up have evaluated the long-term risk for progression to endometrial carcinoma to be less than 5%. [21-23] Furthermore, in patients opting for watchful waiting, spontaneous regression rates of 75% to 100% have been reported. [21,22]

REFERS TO RECOMMENDATION 4

Medical treatment options

There is ample literature supporting the effectiveness of oral progestins and the levonorgestrel-releasing intrauterine system (LNG-IUS) in treating both premenopausal and postmenopausal women with non-atypical endometrial hyperplasia. Disease regression rates for endometrial hyperplasia without atypia of 67% to 72% and 81% to 94% were reported for oral progestins and the LNG-IUS, respectively, in 2 recent meta-analyses including a total of 8 randomized controlled trials. [24-31] Injectable medroxyprogesterone acetate can also be considered as an alternative to the LNG-IUS, with a regression rate reaching 92% at 6 months. [32] The effectiveness and favourable side effect profile of the LNG-IUS make it the treatment of choice for patients with endometrial hyperplasia without atypia. Aromatase inhibitors also represent an effective treatment option for patients with endometrial hyperplasia without atypia. Letrozole had a comparable effectiveness to megestrol acetate and a favourable side effect profile in a recently conducted RCT. [33] They may be used in premenopausal and postmenopausal women. Table 4 offers an overview of progestins used in the conservative treatment of endometrial hyperplasia.

Table 4. Progestins used in the conservative management of endometrial hyperplasia

	Progestin		Trade name	Usual doses
MPA	Oral continuous	High-dose	Provera	100−200 mg/day
		Low-dose		2.5−20 mg/day
	Oral cyclic			10−20 mg/day×10−12 days/cycle
	Injectable		Depo-Provera	150 mg every 90 days
MA	High-dose		Megace	80−320 mg/day
	Low-dose			40 mg/day
NETA	Oral continuous		Norlutate	5−15 mg/day
	Oral cyclic			15 mg/day×10−12 days/cycle
Progesterone			Prometrium	100−300 mg/day
LNG-IUS			Mirena	20 mg/day

LNG-IUS: levonorgestrel intrauterine system; MA: megestrol acetate; MPA: medroxyprogesterone acetate; NETA: norethindrone acetate.

Medical treatment duration and follow-up

A minimum treatment duration of 6 months is usually necessary to induce regression of endometrial hyperplasia without atypia with either oral progestins or the LNG-IUS. [34] Follow-up of treatment response should be done by endometrial sampling, which can be performed with the intrauterine device in place. Endometrial biopsy every 3−6 months is usually performed to ensure that there is no disease progression while on treatment. [5,20] The decision to continue therapy beyond 6 months for patients who do not respond should be made on an individual basis. [35] However, patients who do not respond after 12 months of treatment will rarely show a response thereafter, and a change in treatment modality should be considered. [5] Treatment with progestins is generally continued for 6 months, whereas the LNG-IUS is kept in place for 5 years in patients showing treatment response. [5,36] The relapse rate has proven to be higher in patients treated with progestins and in those with a BMI of 35 kg/m² or greater. [37] The follow-up duration for those patients should therefore be extended. [38]

REFERS TO RECOMMENDATIONS 5 & 6

Indications for surgical treatment

Surgical treatment should be reserved for patients who do not desire to preserve their fertility and who experience progression to atypical hyperplasia or carcinoma during follow-up, whose hyperplasia fails to regress after 12 months of medical treatment or relapses after completing, who continue to experience abnormal uterine bleeding despite treatment, or who decline endometrial surveillance or medical treatment. [39] Surgical management is discussed separately.

REFERS TO RECOMMENDATION 7

Atypical Endometrial Hyperplasia/Endometrial Intraepithelial Neoplasia

Initial management

As up to 60% of patients with EIN already have developed or will develop an invasive endometrial cancer,[7] total hysterectomy with bilateral salpingo—oophorectomy (BSO) is the treatment of choice in patients with this condition. Surgical management is discussed separately.

Medical treatment options and follow-up

Uterine preservation may be considered in patients who wish to preserve their fertility or who are medically unfit for surgery. Counselling is important and should include not only the risk of underlying endometrial malignancy but also the risks of endometrial cancer higher than stage I (2%), coexisting ovarian cancer (4%), and death (0.5%). [40] In a systematic review of uncontrolled studies, those outcomes could not easily be predicted by pre-treatment investigations. [40] Therapeutic goals in fertility preservation include complete reversal of disease, return of the endometrium to its normal function, and prevention of invasive disease; for poor surgical candidates, the goals of medical treatment are disease stabilization and cancer prevention. [41] Conservative treatment options include progestins (oral or local), aromatase inhibitors, or gonadotropin-releasing hormone agonists. Table 4 shows types of progestins and dosages that can be used in treatment of EIN. Again, a trial of 6 months is generally necessary to see a treatment response, with a plateau at around 12 months. [40,42] Regression rates of

55% to 92% and recurrence rates of 3% to 55% have been reported. [33,40,42-45] Metformin may also be added to increase the treatment effect, even in the absence of metabolic syndrome. [46,47] Of note, obesity is associated with a lower chance of disease remission. [43] Endometrial surveillance should be carried out every 3 months until at least 2 negative specimens are obtained. [34,40] The highest risk of disease recurrence being in the first 2 years after treatment cessation, endometrial biopsy every 6 months for 2 years and every year thereafter is recommended until risk factors are corrected or total hysterectomy with BSO is performed. [37,48] Patients who experience progression to carcinoma during follow-up, whose hyperplasia fails to regress after 12 months of medical treatment or relapses after completing treatment with progestins, who continue to experience abnormal uterine bleeding despite treatment, or who decline endometrial surveillance or medical treatment should undergo definitive surgical treatment. [39] In patients who are not surgical candidates, recurrences may be retreated with a second round of progestins with an expected response rate reaching 85% and a possibility of response to a third round of treatment in case of a second recurrence. [49]

Fertility-sparing treatment of endometrial intraepithelial neoplasia

Patients with EIN who wish to preserve their fertility should be referred to a reproductive endocrinologist early as they are at risk of disease recurrence and subfertility. [40] Fertility preservation options include oocyte or embryo cryopreservation prior to hysterectomy with BSO, medical treatment followed by assisted reproductive technology, as well as hysterectomy with ovarian preservation and future use of a surrogate. [50,55] Health care providers should refer these patients to a gynaecologic oncologist as underlying neoplasia is fairly common. [51] Women should be encouraged to maintain a BMI below 30 kg/m^2, as relapse is much more common in obese patients. [51,52] Cancer incidence does not seem to be increased when comparing patients undergoing primary hysterectomy and delayed hysterectomy for fertility-sparing purposes. [53] In fact, infertility treatments do not seem to increase the relapse rate of EIN. [54] The live birth rate associated with conservative management of EIN approximates 7% to 26%, and pregnancy is associated with a lower chance of disease recurrence. [40,42,34,54] The risk of disease recurrence being high, a hysterectomy with BSO is recommended when childbearing is no longer desired. [41,56]

SURGICAL MANAGEMENT

Indications for Surgical Management of Endometrial Hyperplasia Without Atypia

Total hysterectomy for endometrial hyperplasia without atypia offers definitive treatment but is a major surgical procedure with associated morbidity and loss of fertility. In general, hysterectomy is reserved for indications such as persistent or recurrent hyperplasia despite progestin use, progression to atypical hyperplasia or carcinoma, ongoing abnormal uterine bleeding, and patient preference. Surgery would also be appropriate in patients with contraindication or intolerance to medical therapy, an inability or unwillingness to comply with ongoing surveillance, no desire for future fertility, and high baseline risk for endometrial carcinoma. [36,56]

Surgical treatment for endometrial hyperplasia without atypia should consist of total hysterectomy with salpingectomy, with or without bilateral oophorectomy. [39] The ovaries are typically removed in postmenopausal women. However, in premenopausal patients, ovarian preservation should be considered due to the long-term risk of all-cause mortality and morbidity associated with bilateral oophorectomy in young women, particularly in patients under age 45. [57] Prophylactic salpingectomy alone at the time of hysterectomy can be offered for risk reduction of ovarian cancer when the ovaries are left in situ. [58]

REFERS TO SUMMARY STATEMENT 2

Atypical endometrial hyperplasia / endometrial intraepithelial neoplasia

Total hysterectomy with BSO is the preferred treatment for atypical endometrial hyperplasia because of the high risk of progression to malignancy or concurrent endometrial carcinoma. [23,59] Observational studies have reported that an underlying carcinoma is found in up to 60% of endometrial biopsy specimens reported as atypical endometrial hyperplasia. [59-64] For the same reason, it is typically advised that both premenopausal and postmenopausal women undergo BSO in addition to total hysterectomy. The increased risk of mortality and morbidity associated with bilateral oophorectomy in premenopausal women with benign disease should be discussed thoroughly and treatment tailored to each individual. [56]

Surgical approach

There is no evidence to guide the choice of approach for hysterectomy for endometrial hyperplasia without atypia. Given that this pathologic subtype is considered to be a non-neoplastic entity, [64] vaginal, laparoscopic, and open approaches are all acceptable. There are fewer perioperative complications when hysterectomy for benign disease is performed either vaginally or laparoscopically. [6]

Atypical endometrial hyperplasia is associated with higher risk of underlying carcinoma, and therefore the surgical approach should include evaluation of the adnexa and other pelvic structures for signs of invasive disease. Compared with open procedures, laparoscopy leads to fewer perioperative complications, shorter hospital stay, and quicker return to normal activity. [65] Even in cases of endometrial cancer, survival outcomes are similar when surgery is performed by laparoscopy versus by laparotomy. [65] For these reasons, a minimally invasive approach to hysterectomy should be considered first for atypical endometrial hyperplasia, with laparotomy limited to cases where this is not feasible.

Subtotal (supracervical) hysterectomy and morcellation should be avoided in all instances of endometrial hyperplasia due to concern about malignancy and dissemination of disease. [39]

REFERS TO SUMMARY STATEMENTS 3, 4 & 5
REFERS TO RECOMMENDATIONS 8, 9 &10

Other surgical considerations

The literature on the accuracy of frozen section at the time of hysterectomy for endometrial hyperplasia to rule out cancer is inconsistent and limited to small observational studies. [66-72]

There are several reports that favour frozen section intraoperatively to determine which patients require surgical staging for cancer. [68-72] One limitation of this approach is the potential for incongruent results between the frozen section and final pathology, which could result in overtreatment or undertreatment at the time of surgery. [67] Additionally, centres may not have a pathologist in house for frozen section analysis or an available skilled practitioner to perform lymphadenectomy if deemed necessary. If endometrial carcinoma is diagnosed on final pathology after hysterectomy, it is often well differentiated and not associated with high-risk features that require additional surgical staging. [59,66,73] It is reasonable to conduct surgery for endometrial hyperplasia in centres where frozen section is not available. [66] Overall there is not enough evidence to strongly support routine use of frozen section at the time of surgery for endometrial hyperplasia.

REFERS TO SUMMARY STATEMENT 6

Visual inspection

Gross inspection of the uterus by the surgeon is another means to assess depth of myometrial invasion and need for pelvic lymphadenectomy intraoperatively. The available data to support this practice are sparse. [74,75] One should, however, be aware that an inaccurate visual appreciation of the specimen could lead to incorrect surgical decisions. Such practice is not encouraged, as it could damage the specimen and thus interfere with proper pathologic analysis.

Lymphadenectomy

Although there is concern for underlying malignancy in cases of atypical endometrial hyperplasia, surgical staging to include pelvic lymph node dissection would result in overtreatment for the majority of patients. [59,76] When considering the added surgical risk of lymphadenectomy at the time of hysterectomy, more conservative treatment is favoured initially as the chance of a high-risk carcinoma is low. [59,76] A Cochrane review from 2015 did not show evidence to support routine lymphadenectomy for early-stage endometrial cancer[76]; however, practice varies among centres as sentinel lymph node assessment becomes routine practice and replaces full lymph node dissections. Gynaecologic oncology consultation should be obtained to determine management in all cases of endometrial cancer diagnosed on frozen section or final pathology.

REFERS TO SUMMARY STATEMENT 7

Endometrial Ablation

There are reports of endometrial resection and ablation for successful long-term management of endometrial hyperplasia without atypia. [64,77] The largest prospective study included 161 patients who underwent endometrial resection or ablation for simple endometrial hyperplasia and complex hyperplasia without atypia. [64] The median follow-up time was 7 years, and the majority of patients (95.7%) had no further bleeding or pain. Twelve patients went on to have hysterectomy during follow-up, and the final pathology did not show any persistent hyperplasia in any cases. [64] The authors determined that endometrial ablation is a safe option for treatment of endometrial hyperplasia without atypia. [64] One limitation of this technique is the difficulty in confirming complete destruction of the endometrium. Ongoing surveillance can also be challenging due to obliteration of the endometrial cavity, a particular cause for concern in patients with ongoing risk factors for endometrial carcinoma.

There is not sufficient evidence to support endometrial ablation as first-line treatment for endometrial hyperplasia without atypia except in circumstances where major surgery is contraindicated. In cases where the diagnosis is obtained incidentally after completion of endometrial ablation, further treatment may not be necessary, particularly in cases of endometrial resection. [64] Patients should be followed up at regular intervals and investigated if abnormal bleeding persists or recurs.

Endometrial resection or ablation is generally avoided in patients with atypical hyperplasia because it is a pre-malignant condition. Treatment in these cases should be reserved for patients who are poor surgical candidates and in consultation with gynaecology oncology.

REFERS TO SUMMARY STATEMENT 8

Management of Endometrial Hyperplasia Found in an Endometrial Polyp

When endometrial hyperplasia is diagnosed within an endometrial polyp, sampling of the background endometrium is recommended, even when its hysteroscopic appearance is normal. Endometrial hyperplasia either with or without atypia will be found in background endometrium in up to 52% of cases. [78] A systematic review of 10 mostly retrospective studies reported the risk of concurrent endometrial cancer in patients found to have an atypical endometrial polyp to be 5.6%. [79] Endometrial hyperplasia found in endometrial polyps should be treated according to its histologic classification.

REFERS TO SUMMARY STATEMENT 9

REFERENCES

[1] REED S D, NEWTON K M, CLINTON W L, et al. Incidence of endometrial hyperplasia. Am J Obstet Gynecol, 2009, 200: 678, e1-6.

[2] ABU HASHIM H, GHAYATY E, EL RAKHAWY M. Levonorgestrel-releasing intrauterine system vs oral progestins for non-atypical endometrial hyperplasia: a systematic review and meta-analysis of randomized trials. Am J Obstet Gynecol, 2015, 213: 469-478.

[3] EMONS G, BECKMANN M W, SCHMIDT D, et al. New who classification of endometrial hyperplasias. Geburtshilfe Frauenheilkd, 2015, 75: 135 -136.

[4] ZAINO R, CARINELLI S G, ELLENSON L H, et al. WHO Classification of Tumours of Female Reproductive Organs. 4th edition ed. Lyon, France: WHO Press, 2014: 125-126.

[5] MOORE E, SHAFI M. Endometrial hyperplasia. Obstet Gynaecol Reprod Med, 2013, 23: 88-93.

[6] The Cancer Genome Atlas Research NetworkKandoth C, SCHULTZ N, et al. Integrated genomic characterization of endometrial carcinoma. Nature, 2013, 497: 67-73.

[7] ANTONSEN S L, ULRICH L, HOGDALL C. Patients with atypical hyperplasia of the endometrium should be treated in oncological centers. Gynecol Oncol, 2012, 125: 124-128.

[8] CHANDRA V, KIM J J, BENBROOK D M, et al. Therapeutic options for management of endometrial hyperplasia. J Gynecol Oncol, 2016, 27: e8.

[9] FRASER I S, CRITCHLEY H O, BRODER M, et al. The FIGO recommendations on terminologies and definitions for normal and abnormal uterine bleeding. Semin Reprod Med, 2011, 29: 383—390.

[10] PENNANT M E, MEHTA R, MOODY P, et al. Premenopausal abnormal uterine bleeding and risk of endometrial cancer. BJOG, 2017, 124: 404—411.

[11] RENAUD M C, LE T. SOGC-GOC-SCC Policy and Practice Guidelines Committee: Epidemiology and investigations for suspected endometrial cancer. J Obstet Gynaecol Can, 2013, 35: 380—381.

[12] SINGH S, BEST C, DUNN S, et al. Abnormal uterine bleeding in premenopausal women (replaces No. 106, Aug 2001). J Obstet Gynaecol Can, 2013, 35 (5 eSuppl): S1—28.

[13] TRAM S, MUSONDA P, EWIES A A. Premenopausal bleeding: when should the endometrium be investigated? A retrospective non-comparative study of 3006 women. Eur J Obstet Gynecol Reprod Biol, 2010, 148: 86—89.

[14] WISE M R, GILL P, LENSEN S, et al. Body mass index trumps age in decision for endometrial biopsy: cohort study of symptomatic premenopausal women. Am J Obstet Gynecol, 2016, 215. 598. e1—8.

[15] DIJKHUIZEN F P, MOL B W, BROLMANN H A, et al. The accuracy of endometrial sampling in the diagnosis of patients with endometrial carcinoma and hyperplasia. Cancer, 2000, 89: 1765—1772.

[16] SHERMAN M E, RONNETT B, IOOFE O, et al. Reproducibility of biopsy diagnoses of endometrial hyperplasia: evidence supporting a simplified classification. Int J Gynecol Pathol, 2008, 27: 318—325.

[17] WHEELER D T, BRISTOW R E, KURMAN R J. Histologic alterations in endometrial hyperplasia and well-differentiated carcinoma treated with progestins. Am J Surg Pathol, 2007, 31: 988—998.

[18] BEAVIS A L, CHEEMA S, HOLSCHNEIDER C H, et al. Almost

half of women with endometrial cancer or hyperplasia do not know that obesity affects their cancer risk. Gynecol Oncol Rep, 2015, 13: 71-75.

[19] SANGUAKEO A, UPALA S. Bariatric surgery and risk of postoperative endometrial cancer: a systematic review and meta-analysis. Surg Obes Relat Dis, 11: 949-955.

[20] Committee on Gynecologic Practice Society of Gynecologic Oncology. The American College of Obstetricians and Gynecologists committee opinion no. 631. Endometrial intraepithelial neoplasia. Obstet Gynecol, 2015, 125: 1272 -1278.

[21] KURMAN R J, KAMINSKI P F, NORRIS H J. The behavior of endometrial hyperplasia: A long-term study of "untreated" hyperplasia in 170 patients. Cancer, 1985, 56: 403-412.

[22] TERAKAWA N, KIGAWA J, TAKETANI Y, et al. The behavior of endometrial hyperplasia: a prospective study. Endometrial Hyperplasia Study Group. J Obstet Gynaecol Res, 1997, 23: 223-230.

[23] LACEY J V Jr, SHERMAN M E, RUSH B B, et al. Absolute risk of endometrial carcinoma during 20-year follow-up among women with endometrial hyperplasia. J Clin Oncol, 2010, 28: 788-792.

[24] ISMAIL M T, FAHMY D M, ELSHMAA N S. Efficacy of levonorgestrelreleasing intrauterine system versus oral progestins in treatment of simple endometrial hyperplasia without atypia. Reprod Sci, 2013, 20: 45-50.

[25] DOLAPCIOGLU K, BOZ A, BALOGLU A. The efficacy of intrauterine versus oral progestin for the treatment of endometrial hyperplasia: A prospective randomized comparative study. Clin Exp Obstet Gynecol, 2013, 40: 122 -126.

[26] ABU HASHIM H, ZAYED A, GHAYATY E, et al. LNG-IUS treatment of nonatypical endometrial hyperplasia in perimenopausal women: a randomized controlled trial. J Gynecol Oncol, 2013, 24: 128-134.

[27] KARIMI-ZARCHI M, DEHGHANI-FIROOZABADI R, TABA-TABAIE A, et al. A comparison of the effect of levonorgestrel IUD with oral

medroxyprogesterone acetate on abnormal uterine bleeding with simple endometrial hyperplasia and fertility preservation. Clin Exp Obstet Gynecol, 2013, 40: 421—424.

[28] BEHNAMFAR F, GHAHIRI A, TAVAKOLI M. Levonorgestrel-releasing intrauterine system (Mirena) in compare to medroxyprogesterone acetate as a therapy for endometrial hyperplasia. J Res Med Sci, 2014, 19: 686—690.

[29] ORBO A, VEREIDE A B, ARNES M, et al. Levonorgestrel-impregnated intrauterine device as treatment for endometrial hyperplasia: a national multicentre randomised trial. BJOG, 2014, 121: 477—486.

[30] EL BEHERY M M, SALEH H S, IBRAHIEM M A, et al. Levonorgestrel-releasing intrauterine device versus dydrogesterone for management of endometrial hyperplasia without atypia. Reprod Sci, 2015, 22: 329—334.

[31] ABDELAZIZ A M, ABOSRIE M. Levonorgestrel-releasing intrauterine system is an efficient therapeutic modality for simple endometrial hyperplasia. J Am Sci, 2013: 417—424.

[32] NOOH A M, ABDELDAYEM H M, GIRBASH E F, et al. Depo-Provera versus norethisterone acetate in management of endometrial hyperplasia without atypia. Reprod Sci, 2016, 23: 448—454.

[33] MORADAN S, NIKKHAH N, MIRMOHAMMADKHANAI M. Comparing the administration of letrozole and megestrol acetate in the treatment of women with simple endometrial hyperplasia without atypia: a randomized clinical trial. Adv Ther, 2017, 34: 1211—1220.

[34] GUNDERSON C C, FADER A N, CARSON K A, et al. Oncologic and reproductive outcomes with progestin therapy in women with endometrial hyperplasia and grade 1 adenocarcinoma: a systematic review. Gynecol Oncol, 2012, 125: 477—482.

[35] ARMSTRONG A J, HURD W W, ELGUERO S, et al. Diagnosis and management of endometrial hyperplasia. J Minim Invasive Gynecol, 2012, 19: 562—571.

[36] GALLOS I D, SHEHMAR M, THANGARATINAM S, et al. Oral

progestogens vs levonorgestrel-releasing intrauterine systemfor endometrial hyperplasia: A systematic review and metaanalysis. Am J Obstet Gynecol, 2010, 203: 547, e1−10.

[37] GALLOS I D, KRISHAN P, SHEHMAR M, et al. LNG-IUS versus oral progestogen treatment for endometrial hyperplasia: a long-term comparative cohort study. Hum Reprod, 2013, 28: 2966−2971.

[38] GALLOS I D, GANESAN R, GUPTA J K. Prediction of regression and relapse of endometrial hyperplasia with conservative therapy. Obstet Gynecol, 2013, 121: 1165−1171.

[39] GALLOS I D, ALAZZAM M, CLARK T J, et al. Management of endometrial hyperplasia. Green-top guideline No 67. London: Royal College of Obstetricians and Gynaecologists; 2016. Available at: https: // www. rcog. org. uk/globalassets/documents/guidelines/green-top-guidelines/gtg _ 67 _ endometrial _ hyperplasia. pdf. Accessed on April 15, 2019.

[40] GALLOS I D, YAP J, RAJKHOWA M, et al. Regression, relapse, and live birth rates with fertility-sparing therapy for endometrial cancer and atypical complex endometrial hyperplasia: A systematic review and metaanalysis. Am J Obstet Gynecol, 2012, 207: 266, e1−12.

[41] TRIMBLE C L, METHOD M, LEITAO M, et al. Management of endometrial precancers. Obstet Gynecol, 2012, 120: 1160−1175.

[42] SIMPSON A N, FEIGENBERG T, CLARKE B A, et al. Fertility sparing treatment of complex atypical hyperplasia and low grade endometrial cancer using oral progestin. Gynecol Oncol, 2014, 133: 229−233.

[43] CHEN M, JIN Y, LI Y, et al. Oncologic and reproductive outcomes after fertility-sparing management with oral progestin for women with complex endometrial hyperplasia and endometrial cancer. Int J Gynaecol Obstet, 2016, 132: 34−38.

[44] PRONIN S M, NOVIKOVA O V, ANDREEVA J Y, et al. Fertility-sparing treatment of early endometrial cancer and complex atypical hyperplasia in young women of childbearing potential. Int J Gynecol Cancer, 2015, 25: 1010−

1014.

[45] OHYAGI-HARA C, SAWADA K, AKI I, et al. Efficacies and pregnancy outcomes of fertility-sparing treatment with medroxyprogesterone acetate for endometrioid adenocarcinoma and complex atypical hyperplasia: our experience and a review of the literature. Arch Gynecol Obstet, 2015, 291: 151−157.

[46] SHAN W, WANG C, ZHANG Z, et al. Conservative therapy with metformin plus megestrol acetate for endometrial atypical hyperplasia. J Gynecol Oncol, 2014, 25: 214−220.

[47] MITSUHASHI A, SATO Y, KIYOKAWA T, et al. Phase II study of medroxyprogesterone acetate plus metformin as a fertility-sparing treatment for atypical endometrial hyperplasia and endometrial cancer. Ann Oncol, 2016, 27: 262−266.

[48] ORBO A, ARNES M, VEREIDE A B, et al. Relapse risk of endometrial hyperplasia after treatment with the levonorgestrel-impregnated intrauterine system or oral progestogens. BJOG, 2016, 123: 1512−1519.

[49] PARK J Y, LEE S H, SEONG S J, et al. Progestin re-treatment in patients with recurrent endometrial adenocarcinoma after successful fertility-sparing management using progestin. Gynecol Oncol, 2013, 129: 7−11.

[50] KUDESIA R, SINGER T, CAPUTO T A, et al. Reproductive and oncologic outcomes after progestin therapy for endometrial complex atypical hyperplasia or carcinoma. Am J Obstet Gynecol, 2014, 210: 255, e14.

[51] YANG Y F, LIAO Y Y, LIU X L. Prognostic factors of regression and relapse of complex atypical hyperplasia and well-differentiated endometrioid carcinoma with conservative treatment. Gynecol Oncol, 2015, 139: 419−423.

[52] LI M, SONG J L, ZHAO Y, et al. Fertility outcomes in infertile women with complex hyperplasia or complex atypical hyperplasia who received progestin therapy and in vitro fertilization. J Zhejiang Univ Sci B, 2017, 18: 1022−1025.

[53] GONTHIER C, PIEL B, TOUBOUL C, et al. Cancer incidence in patients with atypical endometrial hyperplasia managed by primary hysterectomy or

fertility-sparing treatment. Anticancer Res, 2015, 35: 6799—6804.

[54] ICHINOSE M, FUJIMOTO A, OSUGA Y, et al. The influence of in-fertility treatment on the prognosis of endometrial cancer and atypical complex endometrial hyperplasia. Int J Gynecol Cancer, 2013, 23: 288—293.

[55] GRESSEL G M, PARKASH V, PAL L. Management options and fertility-preserving therapy for premenopausal endometrial hyperplasia and early-stage endometrial cancer. Int J Gynaecol Obstet, 2015, 131: 234—239.

[56] GALLOS I D, KRISHAN P, SHEHMAR M, et al. Relapse of endo-metrial hyperplasia after conservative treatment: a cohort study with long-term follow-up. Hum Reprod, 2013, 28: 1231—1236.

[57] PARKER W H, FESKANICH D, BRODER M S, et al. Long-term mortality associated with oophorectomy compared with ovarian conservation in the Nurses'Health Study. Obstet Gynecol, 2013, 121: 709—716.

[58] SALVADOR S, SCOTT S, FRANCIS J A, et al. No. 344-Opportun-istic salpingectomy and other methods of risk reduction for ovarian/fallopian tube/peritoneal cancer in the general population. J Obstet Gynaecol Can, 2017, 39: 480—493.

[59] TRIMBLE C L, KAUDERER J, ZAINO R, et al. Concurrent endom-etrial carcinoma in women with a biopsy diagnosis of atypical endometrial hyper-plasia: a Gynecologic Oncology Group study. Cancer, 2006, 106: 812—819.

[60] RAKHA E, WONG S C, SOOMRO I, et al. Clinical outcome of atyp-ical endometrial hyperplasia diagnosed on an endometrial biopsy: institutional ex-perience and review of literature. Am J Surg Pathol, 2012, 36: 1683—1690.

[61] WHYTE J S, GURNEY E P, CURTIN J P, et al. Lymph node dis-section in the surgical management of atypical endometrial hyperplasia. Am J Ob-stet Gynecol, 2010, 202: 176, e1—4.

[62] TAŞKIN S, KAN Ö, DAI Ö, et al. Lymph node dissection in atypical endometrial hyperplasia. J Turk Ger Gynecol Assoc, 2017, 18: 127—132.

[63] GIEDE K C, YEN T W, CHIBBAR R, et al. Significance of concur-rent endometrial cancer in women with a preoperative diagnosis of atypical endo-

metrial hyperplasia. J Obstet Gynaecol Can, 2008, 30: 896-901.

[64] VILOS G A, ORAIF A, VILOS A G, et al. Long-term clinical outcomes following resectoscopic endometrial ablation of non-atypical endometrial hyperplasia in women with abnormal uterine bleeding. J Minim Invasive Gynecol, 2015, 22: 66-77.

[65] GALAAL K, BRYANT A, FISHER A D, et al. Laparoscopy versus laparotomy for the management of early stage endometrial cancer. Cochrane Database Syst Rev, 2012, 9: CD006655.

[66] BOYRAZ G, BAŞARAN D, SALMAN M C, et al. Does preoperative diagnosis of endometrial hyperplasia necessitate intraoperative frozen section consultation? Balkan Med J, 2016, 33: 657-661.

[67] INDERMAUR M D, SHOUP B, TEBES S, et al. The accuracy of frozen pathology at time of hysterectomy in patients with complex atypical hyperplasia on preoperative biopsy. Am J Obstet Gynecol, 2007, 196: e40-42.

[68] MOROTTI M, MENADA M V, MOIOLI M, et al. Frozen section pathology at time of hysterectomy accurately predicts endometrial cancer in patients with preoperative diagnosis of atypical endometrial hyperplasia. Gynecol Oncol, 2012, 125: 536-540.

[69] STEPHAN J M, HANSEN J, SAMUELSON M, et al. Intra-operative frozen section results reliably predict final pathology in endometrial cancer. Gynecol Oncol, 2014, 133: 499-505.

[70] MONTALTO S A, COUTTS M, DEVAJA O, et al. Accuracy of frozen section diagnosis at surgery in pre-malignant and malignant lesions of the endometrium. Eur J Gynaecol Oncol, 2008, 29 (5): 435-440.

[71] OZ M, OZGU E, KORKMAZ E, et al. Utility of frozen section pathology with endometrial pre-malignant lesions. Asian Pac J Cancer Prev, 2014, 15: 6053-6057.

[72] SALMAN M C, USUBUTUN A, DOGAN N U, et al. The accuracy of frozen section analysis at hysterectomy in patients with atypical endometrial hyperplasia. Clin Exp Obstet Gynecol, 2009, 36 (1): 31-34.

[73] ODA K, KOGA K, HIRATA T, et al. Risk of endometrial cancer in patients with a preoperative diagnosis of atypical endometrial hyperplasia treated with total laparoscopic hysterectomy. Gynecol Minim Invasive Ther, 2016, 5: 69—73.

[74] MARCICKIEWICZ J, SUNFELDT K. Accuracy of intraoperative gross visual assessment of myometrial invasion in endometrial cancer. Acta Obstet Gynecol Scand, 2011, 90: 846—851.

[75] TRAEN K, HOLUND B, MOGENSEN O. Accuracy of preoperative tumor grade and intraoperative gross examination of myometrial invasion in patients with endometrial cancer. Acta Obstet Gynecol Scand, 2007, 86: 739 —741.

[76] FROST J A, WEBSTER K E, BRYANT A, et al. Lymphadenectomy for the management of endometrial cancer. Cochrane Database Syst Rev, 2015, 9: CD007585.

[77] AVCI M E, SADIK S, UÇCAR M G. A prospective study of rollerball endometrial ablation in the management of refractory recurrent symptomatic endometrial hyperplasia without atypia. Gynecol Obstet Investig, 2012, 74: 282— 287.

[78] KELLY P, DOBBS S P, MCCLUGGAGE W G. Endometrial hyperplasia involving endometrial polyps: Report of a series and discussion of the significance in an endometrial biopsy specimen. BJOG, 2007, 114: 944—950.

[79] DE RIJK S R, STEENBERGEN M E, NIEBOER T E, et al. Atypical endometrial polyps and concurrent endometrial cancer: a systematic review. Obstet Gynecol, 2016, 128: 519—525.

附录 D　ISGE 指南——宫腔镜子宫肌瘤切除

　　子宫黏膜下肌瘤占所有子宫肌瘤的 5.5%～10%，在 50 岁时患病率高达 70%～80%[1]。其在美国每年的经济成本超过乳腺癌、卵巢癌和结肠癌[2,3]。突入宫腔的子宫黏膜下肌瘤，可能会在月经期诱发大量子宫出血以及剧烈痛经，也易使患者不孕[4]。宫腔镜下子宫肌瘤去除术（hysteroscopic myomectomy，HM）是子宫黏膜下肌瘤的一线微创保守手术治疗方式，适用于尚未完成生育的女性。国际妇科内镜学会（International Society for Gynecologic Endoscopy，ISGE）旨在从目前可用于 HM 的最佳证据中为临床医生提供推荐建议。

一、材料和方法

　　国际妇科内镜学会 HM 工作组总结了与宫腔镜下子宫肌瘤去除术相关的重点临床问题（附表 D-1），据此在 Medline、PubMed 以及 Cochrane 数据库中进行了搜索。我们收集并分析了自 2005 年 1 月至 2021 年 6 月发表过的相关英文文献，包括原始著作、综述、欧洲妇科内镜学会（European Society for Gynecological Endoscopy，ESGE）和美国妇科腹腔镜协会（American Association of Gynecologic Laparoscopists，AAGL）发表过的相关指南。依据 GRADE 评价系统（http://www. gradewor-kinggroup. org；见附表 D-2），针对每一个临床问题，我们将可用信息根据证据等级进行了分级，并且在多轮文献分析及专家讨论的基础上提出推荐建议。经 ISGE 伦理委员会裁定，本研究不需要进行伦理审批。

附表 D-1　宫腔镜下子宫肌瘤去除术关键临床问题

序号	问题
问题 1	HM 术前如何评估患者？
问题 2	依据手术结果进行分类，哪种是子宫黏膜下肌瘤的最佳分类方案？
问题 3	术前药物治疗是否有适应证？
问题 4	0 型子宫黏膜下肌瘤最适合的去除技术和器械是哪种？
问题 5	1 型和 2 型 LM 最适合的切除技术和器械是哪种？
问题 6	哪些措施可以降低 HM 的术中穿孔率？

续表

序号	问题
问题 7	哪些措施可以减少 HM 术中及术后的出血？
问题 8	对于液体不足应该考虑哪些限制？哪些措施可以减低膨宫液相关并发症的发生率？
问题 9	哪些措施可以减少宫颈创伤、感染和粘连？

注：HM，宫腔镜子宫肌瘤去除术；LM，子宫肌瘤。

附表 D-2　GRADE 方法建议分级、风险/收益和支持证据的质量

推荐等级	风险/收益	证据质量
1A. 强烈推荐，高质量	收益明显大于风险和负担，反之亦然	来自科学的随机对照试验或其他形式的压倒性证据的一致性证据。进一步的研究不太可能改变我们对收益和风险估计的信心。
1B. 强烈推荐，中等质量	收益明显大于风险和负担，反之亦然	来自具有重要局限性的随机对照试验的证据（结果不一致，方法学缺陷，间接或不精确），或其他一些研究设计的非常有力的证据。进一步的研究（如果进行）可能会影响我们对收益和风险估计的信心，并可能改变估计。
1C. 强烈推荐，低质量	收益似乎大于风险和负担，反之亦然	来自观察性研究、非系统性临床经验或存在严重缺陷的随机对照试验的证据。任何对效果的估计都是不确定的
2A. 不建议，高质量	收益与风险和负担相当	来自科学的随机对照试验或其他形式的压倒性证据的一致性证据。进一步的研究不太可能改变我们对收益和风险估计的信心。
2B. 不建议，中等治疗	收益与风险和负担相当，在收益、风险和负担的估计中有些不确定	来自具有重要局限性的随机对照试验的证据（结果不一致，方法学缺陷，间接或不精确），或其他一些研究设计的非常有力的证据。进一步的研究（如果进行）可能会影响我们对收益和风险估计的信心，并可能改变估计。
2C. 不建议，低质量	收益、风险和负担估计存在不确定性；收益可能与风险和负担相当	来自观察性研究、非系统性临床经验或存在严重缺陷的随机对照试验的证据。任何对效果的估计都是不确定的。

二、结果和讨论（文献综述，思考分析，推荐建议）

术前评估

临床上，出现异常子宫出血时可怀疑是否存在子宫黏膜下肌瘤，可进一步通过影像学检查进行诊断。影像学检查包括超声（ultrasonography，US）、生理盐水灌注子宫超声显像（saline infusion sonohysterography，SIS）、磁共振成像（magnetic resonance imaging，MRI）和/或诊断性宫腔镜检查[1,2,4]。通过组织学检查可确认最终诊断[5]。全面评估患者和子宫肌层病变的详细特征，旨在确定HM的合适候选人，评估手术风险，减少并发症，并有助于手术的成功完成。对既往资料进行采集和分析，进行体格检查，妊娠和妇科恶性疾病（宫颈癌及内膜癌）患者根据指南应被排除在外[6]，对子宫进行充分评估。术前子宫评估的目的是：确定所有子宫病变，确定子宫黏膜下肌瘤的数量、位置、大小、肌层穿透情况及结节与浆膜之间的最小距离，将子宫肌瘤与子宫其他疾病进行鉴别（如子宫腺肌瘤）。

超声因其实用性、可靠性和成本效益[7]，是评估子宫肌层的首选影像学检查手段。2015 年，国际子宫形态学超声评估（Morphological Uterus Sonographic Assessment，MUSA）小组发表了超声下子宫肌层病变描述术语共识，其中就术语、定义和测量方法进行了统一。这些术语、定义和测量方法可用于描述和报告正常和病理性子宫肌层相关的超声检查结果[8,9]。根据 Pereira 等人的研究（2021），以宫腔镜检查为金标准评价经阴道超声诊断宫内病变的准确性，诊断子宫肌瘤的敏感性为 46.7%，特异性为 95.0%，准确率为 87.9%，Kappa 指数为 0.46[10]。

高质量的证据支持 SIS 在诊断子宫黏膜下肌瘤方面与宫腔镜同样有效，SIS和宫腔镜检查均优于经阴道超声检查[11,12]。在评估子宫肌瘤凸向宫腔及穿透肌层的范围上，SIS 可以提供的信息与宫腔镜检查联合经阴道超声所提供的信息相当。

在子宫肌瘤的诊断上，Stamatopoulos 等人研究表明，MRI 的敏感性为94.1%，特异性为 68.7%，阳性预测值为 95.7%，阴性预测值为 61.1%[14]。MRI 在提供有关子宫黏膜下肌瘤的准确信息方面被认为优于其他技术[7,14-17]，但对所有患者常规使用并不具有成本效益。对于体重指数高、肌瘤数量多、子宫体积大、同时存在其他子宫或盆腔病变的患者，可以进行 MRI 检查[7]。MRI 和超声在诊断子宫腺肌病/腺肌瘤方面具有相同的特异性，但比超声具有更高的敏感性[1,18]，由于治疗策略不同，应在术前将子宫腺肌病/腺肌瘤与子宫肌瘤区分开来。当超声指示非典型病变时，增强 MRI 检查适合用来对子宫肌层恶性肿瘤可能性大小进行术前评估[5]。据报道，接受宫腔镜手术的患者中子宫肉瘤的发生率为 0.13%[19,20]。

CT、CT 仿真宫腔镜检查和子宫输卵管造影因为不能提供准确的信息，很少用于拟行 HM 的患者。

门诊宫腔镜检查可以直观地观察子宫腔，判断子宫内膜性状，判断是否存在子宫黏膜下肌瘤和其他宫腔内的病变。除了可视外，还可以进行子宫内膜及可视病变活检。Dueholm 等人发现宫腔镜，SIS 和 MRI 对于判断子宫腔内病变的特征上同样有效并优于经阴道超声[15]。为了正确判断肌瘤穿透子宫肌层的深度，门诊宫腔镜检查的同时应联合经阴道超声。这种联合诊断策略不仅代表了一种充分和值得推荐的术前评估方式，而且在可行的情况下，还代表了一种即诊即治的方法[4]。

【推荐建议 1】拟行 HM 患者的术前评估应从详细的病史采集和体格检查开始（推荐等级 1A）。

【推荐建议 2】所有子宫肌瘤患者均应行超声检查（推荐等级 1A），推荐在描述超声检查结果时使用 MUSA 中的术语、定义及测量方法（推荐等级 1B）。

【推荐建议 3】拟行 HM 前，推荐行 SIS 或结合经阴道超声及诊断性宫腔镜检查评估子宫情况（推荐等级 1A）。当超声评估存在局限性时（如患者体重指数高、肌瘤数量多、子宫体积大、同时存在其他子宫或盆腔病变、子宫肿瘤性质不明确），可以使用 MRI 检查进行评估（推荐等级 1A）。

【推荐建议 4】术前必须给予患者适当的知情同意，解释替代治疗方案、HM 的潜在风险、二次干预以及子宫肌瘤复发的可能性。

三、子宫黏膜下肌瘤的分类

对子宫肌瘤进行恰当的分类对于指导治疗方案选择，包括手术方案选择具有重要意义。Ricardo Lasmar 提出了所谓的 STEPW 分类[24]，基于对五个子宫黏膜下肌瘤特征进行打分：大小、形态、基底延伸、穿透范围和侧壁位置（附表 D

—3）。前瞻性多中心研究表明，与 ESGE 先前提出的分类系统相比，STEPW 分类可以更好地预测复杂 HM、手术时间、肌瘤切除不完整、液体平衡、并发症的发生率和严重程度[25,26]。由于 HM 可能需要两次或更多次手术才可完成，STEPW 评分系统能够比仅基于子宫肌瘤大小和肌壁穿透程度的估计更好地预测两次或更多次手术的风险[27-29]。

附表 D-3　黏膜下肌瘤的 STEPW 分类

分数/分	大小	形态	基底延伸	穿透范围	侧壁位置
0	<2 cm	低	<1/3	0	+1
1	2~5 cm	中	1/3~2/3	<50%	
2	>5 cm	高	>2/3	>50%	
得分					
0~4	第一组	低复杂度 HM			
5~6	第二组	高复杂度 HM，分词 HM，GnRH-a 使用			
7~9	第三组	考虑替代 HM			

注：GnRH-a，促性腺激素释放激素；HM，宫腔镜子宫肌瘤去除术。

【推荐建议 5】推荐使用 STEPW 子宫黏膜下肌瘤分类系统来预测复杂手术、肌瘤切除不完整、手术时间长、液体超载和其他主要并发症的发生（推荐等级 1B）。

四、术前处理

促性腺激素释放激素（gonadotropin-releasing hormone，GnRH）类似物已被用于术前缩小子宫肌瘤大小，减少血管化，目的是加快手术[32,33]。GnRH 诱导低雌激素状态，使子宫肌瘤缩小，但也有副作用，如潮热和盗汗。结合激素反向添加治疗，可以尽可能减少包括骨质丢失在内的低雌激素相关副作用[34]。在最近的一项围绕术前应用 GnRH 的系统综述和荟萃分析中，对以下内容进行了研究：黏膜下肌瘤的完全切除、手术时间、液体吸收以及术中大出血、子宫穿孔和肠损伤等并发症的发生情况[32]。没有发现在 HM 之前给予 GnRH 存在优势。

关于在 HM 前应用醋酸乌利司他（ulipristal acetate，UPA）的作用存在低质量证据[35]。整个欧盟暂停了 UPA 对子宫肌瘤的治疗，等待欧洲药品管理局

(European Medicines Agency，EMA）完成正在进行的对其肝毒性的审查[36]。2020 年 11 月 12 日，EMA 人类药物委员会（CHMP）建议限制使用含有醋酸乌利司他 5 mg 的药物。在等待手术治疗期间，这些药物不得用于控制子宫肌瘤的症状。

【推荐建议 6】不常规推荐术前使用 GnRH 类似物，因为它在促进完整切除黏膜下肌瘤、减少手术时间和液体吸收以及避免重大并发症方面没有被证明是有效的（推荐等级 2B）。

五、0 型子宫肌瘤

HM 的主要目标是完整切除黏膜下肌瘤，保证子宫的解剖完整性。手术宫腔镜是在直接和持续可视控制下进行子宫黏膜下肌瘤去除术的器械。它包括一个带有透镜（0°－12°－30°）的内镜，以及外径为 1～27 French（Fr）的内鞘及外鞘。内外鞘可提供膨宫液的持续流入和流出，以维持持续和有效的宫腔灌洗系统。手术宫腔镜可以使用以下工作元件：电外科器械（电切环、气化电极及激光器）和冷刀器械（剪刀、钳子、冷刀环）来进行传统宫腔镜手术或门诊宫腔镜手术。小直径门诊器械可以通过标准宫腔镜（12～15Fr）的操作通道（5Fr）对小肌瘤进行去除。

根据所使用的器械不同，可应用不同技术进行宫腔镜下 0 型子宫肌瘤切除，如对肌瘤进行电切、粉碎、门诊宫腔镜下剪断肌瘤蒂[4,37]。传统宫腔镜下切除宫腔内肌瘤应用电切技术，由切割环对病变进行重复渐进的操作。通常从肌瘤顶端进行切割，匀速切割至其底部。切割环起于病变远端，回拉进鞘。

虽然电切技术通常被认为是 0 型子宫肌瘤去除术的金标准，但文献中没有确凿的证据支持其优于其他技术[38]。使用宫腔镜组织切除系统进行子宫内粉碎术（Intra Uterine Morcellation，IUM）与电切镜电切术在数量有限的研究中进行了比较，通常是在子宫肌瘤和息肉间进行。IUM 在手术时间和学习曲线方面被证明是更优越的。一项随机对照试验报道，与电切术相比，住院医师在进行粉碎术培训时学习曲线更短[40]。一篇评估 IUM 在处理黏膜下肌瘤可行性的系统综述中表示，不同于 2 型子宫肌瘤，对于 0 型和 1 型子宫肌瘤 IUM 是可行的[41]。然而，这篇综述中的研究提供的证据是非常有限的。一旦黏膜下肌瘤完全暴露在宫腔内，就可以使用 IUM 移除。对于小的带蒂肌瘤，可以考虑进行门诊子宫肌瘤去除术。

【推荐建议 7】对于 0 型子宫肌瘤，除了电切镜（电切技术）外，推荐粉碎术。相对于电切镜，粉碎术术程更快，学习曲线更短（推荐等级 1C）。

六、1 型和 2 型子宫肌瘤

（一）电切技术与粉碎术

目前，缺乏高质量的数据表明切除 1 型或 2 型子宫肌瘤最适合的技术和工具。然而电切技术是可行的并可重复的[1]，大多数分析宫内粉碎术的文献没有区分子宫肌瘤和宫内其他病变。2017 年，Vitale 等人确实发表了一篇关于宫腔镜下黏膜下肌瘤粉碎术的综述[41]。作者分析了 8 项前瞻性随机、非随机和回顾性研究，但未能提供关于 1 型、2 型子宫肌瘤专用粉碎器的结论性信息。出于这个原因，在出现新的高质量研究和数据之前，推荐使用电切技术，因为它是可行的和可重复的。目前，还没有关于比较这两种技术安全性的数据。

（二）电切术——冷刀与热刀

由 Ivan Mazzon 博士首次提出和描述的冷刀技术，在热量扩散到周围组织（即健康子宫内膜和子宫肌层）的风险方面，被认为比电切技术具有更小的侵犯性[42]。然而，当在正确的平面（假包膜）内进行子宫肌瘤去除术时，即使是在 2 型子宫肌瘤的情况下，副损伤也十分有限。

在子宫肌瘤去除术中要避免的主要并发症是血管渗透综合征。文献中没有高质量的信息准确估计由冷刀技术完成的子宫肌瘤去除术患者的血管渗透率。

大多数关注冷刀技术的研究是回顾性或队列研究，由同一组研究人员/外科医生实施[42,43]。从未通过随机对照试验对该技术在生育率或妊娠结局方面的理论优势进行研究。

由于上面提到的一系列原因，目前还没有关于冷刀或电切优越性的相关推荐建议。

（三）电切术——单极与双极

一项唯一的小型随机对照试验比较使用单极或双极进行子宫肌瘤去除术治疗月经过多的不孕妇女[44]。在两组中，均观察到子宫肌瘤去除术后月经症状的显著改善。妊娠相关的结局也是相似的。总之，在缓解症状和改善生育结局方面，使用单极或双极切除没有明确差异。

（四）替换技术

水按摩和双手按摩子宫的方法是为了将肌壁间的子宫肌瘤挤压进入宫腔，进而减少病变切除不完整的风险。一项前瞻性研究[45]对这两种方法进行了评估。这种技术可能很有趣，但随机对照试验对证明其可靠性是必要的。

Tanvir 等人在一项小型前瞻性多中心研究中指出，门诊宫腔镜下子宫肌瘤去除术后将黏膜下肌瘤留在子宫腔内可作为处理小的 0～1 型子宫肌瘤（1，2－2，5 cm）的一种选择，成功率为 89％。这种技术的建立还需要进行更大规模的研究[46]。

可以考虑术中超声引导。根据一些作者的观点，可以使用经腹探头或经直肠探头。这种方法可能有助于一步切除子宫肌瘤和/或避免并发症，如子宫穿孔[47,48]。

【推荐建议 8】对于 1～2 型子宫肌瘤，目前推荐使用电切技术，仅就粉碎术而言，电切技术是可行和可重复的（推荐等级 1C 级）。

【推荐建议 9】对于 1～2 型子宫肌瘤去除术术中使用冷刀或电切的选择，没有可以提出的推荐建议（推荐等级 2C）。

【推荐建议 10】使用单极或双极进行 1～2 型子宫肌瘤去除术在缓解月经症状和生育结局方面作用相当（推荐等级 2B）。

七、HM 的主要特殊并发症及预防措施

（一）宫颈损伤及宫颈/子宫穿孔

宫腔镜手术并发症的发生率（附表 D-4），主要取决于手术的难度，所使用的设备/技术，外科医生的专业技能和患者的个体差异[49]。所有并发症中约有一半是所谓的"进入相关"——宫颈损伤和宫颈或子宫穿孔。风险因素包括解剖变异（极度前倾或后倾）和由于未产、绝经后、剖宫产或切除转化区而导致的宫颈管狭窄。

附表 D-4　宫腔镜手术并发症

并发症	发病率/%
需要输血和止血干预的出血	0.00~0.16
子宫穿孔	0.12~3.00
感染	0.01~1.42
液体过吸收综合征（使用等渗溶液）	
轻度（吸收 1000~2000 mL）	5.0~10.00
重度（吸收>2000 mL）	<1
宫腔粘连	未知
多发性与单发性肌瘤切除的对比	45.50∶31.30*

* 基于有限数量研究案例的资料。

穿孔可能发生在宫颈扩张，放置宫腔镜/电切镜或肌瘤去除术术中。较短的子宫肌瘤与浆膜层间的距离（即子宫肌层游离边缘）是一个重要的危险因素。当激活电极发生穿孔时，相邻解剖结构受损的风险很高。有时候，即使没有穿孔，手术后几天也可能发现相邻器官的迟发热损伤[50]。

在大多数钝性穿孔的病例中，观察和使用抗生素的保守治疗是足够的。然而，在"热能穿孔"的情况下，必须进行腹腔镜（或开腹）探查，以充分评估和治疗可能损害的邻近解剖结构[50]。

关于在宫腔镜检查前经阴道或口服米索前列醇的益处，不同的研究给出了相互矛盾的结果。作为一种促进宫颈成熟的药物，有利于宫颈扩张和宫腔镜放置[51-53]。尽管其使用似乎很有前景[51,52]，但在得出结论之前还需要进一步地研究。

【推荐建议 11】为了减少宫颈损伤和穿孔的发生，不常规推荐在 HM 前经阴道使用米索前列醇（推荐等级 2B 级）。

（二）膨宫液相关并发症

为了达到诊断和治疗宫内病变所必需的可视化，需要用膨宫介质扩张宫腔。在宫腔镜手术过程中，可能发生大量膨宫液的全身吸收，导致严重的并发症（附表 D-4）。吸收量以及患者发病率，例如心血管或肾脏疾病，决定了出现的症状和并发症的严重程度。液体超负荷可导致心力衰竭、肺水肿、低钠血症和脑水肿伴癫痫发作，昏迷和呼吸骤停。持续和准确地监测全身吸收量，即所谓的"体液损失"，对于预防并发症的发生至关重要[54]。

由于液体过吸收性渗透压失衡，使用生理盐水或低渗、非导电、低黏度液体（甘氨酸、山梨醇或甘露醇）可能导致液体过载，导致额外的低渗、低钠血症和低钾血症，需要包括麻醉医师和重症监护医师在内的多学科参与诊疗[55]。

Dyrbye 等人发现，在用盐水溶液进行双极治疗过程中，血管内渗透超过1000 mL 与更严重的气体栓塞发生有关[56]。然而，这种关联并不是因果关系，导致气体栓塞的原因是双极电能产生大量气泡，而不在于膨宫液的吸收量。在双极电切过程中，电子从主动电极移动到被动电极，只有几毫米远；膨宫介质的加热非常强烈，造成"气泡"的产生。在单极电切过程中，电能穿过液体和患者的身体，导致热量降低，因此产生较少的"气泡"。降低双极切除功率，可以减少热量的产生，在血管内吸收等量液体的前提下形成较少的"气泡"，减少栓塞的发生率。这就是在以生理盐水为介质的膨宫液中，使用具有相同功率的小宫腔镜与大宫腔镜，会产生相同数量的"气泡"和气体栓塞的原因。

此外，电切会产生包括一氧化碳在内的废物。使用双极电切时，一氧化碳可能通过液体渗透进入循环，导致碳氧血红蛋白的形成[57,58]。碳氧血红蛋白水平与最大ST 段改变及血管内渗透量之间存在统计学的显著相关性。这种情况会导致心肌缺血。麻醉医师必须参与并发症的处理。出现心电图变化时应该立即停止手术。

【推荐建议 12】育龄期的健康女性在使用双极进行以生理盐水为膨宫介质的宫腔镜下子宫肌瘤去除术中，液体负欠量 1000 mL 时，主要并发症的发生风险较低。液体负欠量 1000～2500 mL 时需要进行严密监测，在出现可能发生栓塞的细微征象时停止手术。液体负欠量超过 2500 mL 时需要立即终止手术（推荐等级 1C 级）。

【推荐建议 13】对于老年人以及患有心血管、肾脏或其他合并症的女性液体负欠量阈值应降低至 750 mL（推荐等级 1B）。

（三）感染

宫腔镜手术后的感染率非常低（附表 D-4）。在未来进行随机高质量试验研究之前，无法得出需要常规抗生素预防用药的结论[59]。

（四）粘连

HM 可能并发严重程度不一的术后子宫腔粘连（intrauterine adhesions, IUA）。对此，为达到一级预防已研制出了各种防粘连凝胶，自交联透明质酸凝胶治疗的患者术后粘连发生率与未接受治疗组相比降低[60,61]。

可以考虑进行门诊二次宫腔镜检查，尤其是对于有生育问题的患者，可以对子宫腔粘连进行诊断并及时去除新形成子宫腔粘连[62]。

【推荐建议 14】HM 后推荐常规应用交联透明质酸凝胶，特别针对多发子宫肌瘤去除术（推荐等级 1B）。

附表 D-5　ISGE 建议的证据来源

推荐	资料来源（参考文献）
术前评估	
推荐建议 1	1，4
推荐建议 2	1，7—10
推荐建议 3	5，11—13，15—17
推荐建议 4	1，4
黏膜下平滑肌瘤的分类	
推荐建议 5	24—26
术前处理	
推荐建议 6	32，33
宫腔镜子宫肌瘤去除术：0 型子宫肌瘤	
推荐建议 7	40，41
宫腔镜子宫肌瘤去除术：1 型和 2 型子宫肌瘤	
推荐建议 8	1，41
推荐建议 9	42，43
推荐建议 10	44
并发症及预防措施	
推荐建议 11	51—53
推荐建议 12 及 13	54—58
推荐建议 14	60，61

注：针对 Meta 分析、指南和综述，对这些出版物的参考文献列表进行了分析，并对引用的相关论文进行了评估。

八、结论

HM 是黏膜下肌瘤最有效的保守性妇科微创治疗。强烈建议应用经阴道超声、诊断性宫腔镜检查或 SIS 联合评估子宫，并应用 STEPW 黏膜下肌瘤分类方案，以预测手术难度或手术完成度及主要并发症发生的可能性。对于 0 型子宫肌瘤，除了经典的宫腔镜电切技术之外，还推荐进行粉碎术，手术速度更快，学习曲线更短。相反，对于 1 型和 2 型子宫肌瘤，推荐使用电切技术，相较粉碎术更有可行和可重复性。预防并发症的意识和护理是至关重要的，特别是连续和准确地计算吸收的膨宫液的负欠量。

在所有 HM（不仅在使用低张膨宫液及单极进行的子宫肌瘤去除术中，而且在使用生理盐水溶液作为膨宫液及双极进行的子宫肌瘤去除术中）中，应将液体负欠量 1 L 作为安全限度。对于老年人以及患有合并症的女性应选择较低的液体负欠量阈值（750 mL）。本文提出的以循证为基础的 ISGE 推荐建议旨在通过促进良好的临床实践和住院医师的培训质量来提高患者的诊治安全。

九、竞争利益声明

作者声明，他们没有已知的可能影响本文所述工作的经济利益竞争或个人关系。

［注］参考文献见英文版。

廖柯鑫　冯力民

Hysteroscopic myomectomy: The guidelines of the International Society for Gynecologic Endoscopy (ISGE)

Introduction

Submucosal leiomyomas (LMs), myomas or fibroids represent 5.5−10% of all uterine LMs which have a prevalence as high as 70−80% at the age of 50[1] and cost annually, in the USA, more than breast, ovarian and colon cancer[2,3]. Protruding into the uterine cavity, submucosal LMs may induce excessive uterine bleeding, usually during menses, and colicky dysmenorrhea, being also thought to predispose patients to reproductive failure[4]. Hysteroscopic myomectomy (HM) is the first-line minimally invasive and conservative surgical treatment for submucosal LMs, thus appropriate in women that have not completed their reproductive path. With this publication, the ISGE aims to provide the clinicians with the recommendations arising from the best evidence currently available on HM.

Material and methods

The ISGE Task Force for HM defined key clinical questions (Table 1), which led the search of Medline/PubMed and the Cochrane Database. We selected and analyzed relevant English-language articles, published from January 2005 to June 2021, including original works, reviews and the guidelines previously published by the European Society for Gynecological Endoscopy (ESGE) and the American Association of Gynecologic Laparoscopists (AAGL). Using the GRADE approach (http://www. gradewor-kinggroup.org; Table 2), we graded the available information by the level of evidence for each clinical question and developed the recommendations through multiple cycles of literature analysis and expert discussion. The ISGE Ethical Committee ruled that approval was not required for this study.

Table 1

Hysteroscopic myomectomy-key clinical questions.

Question 1:	How should a patient be evaluated before HM?
Question 2:	Which is the best classification system for submucous LMs in relation to the surgical outcome?
Question 3:	Are there any indications for preoperative medical treatment?
Question 4:	What is the best resection technique and what are the most suitable instruments for resection of type 0 submucosal LMs?
Question 5:	What is the best resection technique and what are the most suitable instruments for resection of type 1 and type 2 LMs?
Question 6:	Which measures can reduce the perforation rate in HM?
Question 7:	Which measures can reduce bleeding during and after HM?
Question 8:	Which limit should be considered for fluid deficit and which measures cam reduce the rate of distention fluid—related complications?
Question 9:	Which measures can reduce cervical trauma, infections and adhesions?

Abbreviation: HM, hysteroscopic myomectomy; LMs, leiomyomas.

Table 2

GRADE approach-grading of recommendations, risk/benefit and quality of supporting evidence.

Grade of recommendation	Risk/benefit	Quality of supporting evidence
1A. Strong recommendation, high quality evidence	Benefits clearly outweigh risk and burdens, or vice versa.	Consistent evidence from well performed randomized, controlled trials or overwhelming evidence of some other form. Further research is unlikely to change our confidence in the estimate of benefit and risk.
1B. Strong recommendation, moderate quality evidence	Benefits clearly outweigh risk and burdens, or vice versa.	Evidence from randomized, controlled trials with important limitations (inconsistent results, methodologic flaws, indirect or imprecise), or very strong evidence of some other research design. Further research (if performed) is likely to have an impact on our confidence in the estimate of benefit and risk and may change the estimate.
1C. Strong recommendation, low quality evidence	Benefits appear to outweigh risk and burdens, or vice versa.	Evidence from observational studies, unsystematic clinical experience, or from randomized, controlled trials with serious flaws. Any estimate of effect is uncertain.
2A. Weak recommendation, high quality evidence	Benefits closely balanced with risks and burdens.	Consistent evidence from well performed randomized, controlled trials or overwhelming evidence of some other form. Further research is unlikely to change our confidence in the estimate of benefit and risk.
2B. Weak recommendation, moderate quality evidence	Benefits closely balanced with risks and burdens, some uncertainly in the estimates of benefits, risks and burdens.	Evidence from randomized, controlled trials with important limitations (inconsistent results, methodologic flaws, indirect or imprecise), or very strong evidence of some other research design. Further research (if performed) is likely to have an impact on our confidence in the estimate of benefit and risk and may change the estimate.
2C. Weak recommendation, low quality evidence	Uncertainty in the estimates of benefits, risks, and burdens; benefits may be closely balanced with risks and burdens.	Evidence from observational studies, unsystematic clinical experience, or from randomized, controlled trials with serious flaws. Any estimate of effect is uncertain.

Results and discussion

Literature review, considerations and recommendations

Preoperative evaluation

Submucous LMs are clinically suspected by abnormal uterine bleeding (AUB), while the diagnosis is generally established by imaging techniques-ultrasonography (US), saline infusion sonohysterography (SIS), magnetic resonance imaging (MRI), and/or by diagnostic hysteroscopy[1,2,4]. Histological confirmation provides the final diagnosis[5]. Detailed characterization of the patient and thorough characterization of the myometrial lesion (s) aim to identify the right candidate for HM and assess the surgical risks, reduce the complications and contribute to the successful completion of the surgery.

Anamnestic data should be taken and analyzed, physical examination performed, pregnancy and gynecological malignancy (cervical and endometrial cancer) excluded in accordance with the guidelines[6], and adequate uterine evaluation accomplished. The objectives of preoperative uterine assessment are: to identify all uterine lesions; to confirm the number and submucous location and position of LMs, size, myometrial penetration and minimal distance between the nodule and serosa for each identified submucous LM; to distinguish LMs from other uterine lesions (e. g. , adenomyomas).

US is the first-line imaging tool for assessing the myometrium because of its availability, reliability and cost-effectiveness[7]. The Morphological Uterus Sonographic Assessment (MUSA) paper from 2015 provides a consensus statement on terms, definitions and measurements that can be used to describe and report normal and pathological myometrial findings during an ultrasound examination[8,9]. In accordance with the study of Pereira et al. (2021) that evaluated the accuracy of transvaginal US (TVUS) in the diagnosis of intrauterine lesions using hysteroscopy as the gold standard, sensitivity for LMs was 46. 7%, specificity 95. 0%, accuracy 87. 9% and Kappa index 0. 46[10].

High-quality evidence supports that SIS is equally performant as hysteroscopy to diagnose submucous LMs, being both SIS and hysteroscopy superior to TVUS[11,12]. By defining the extent to which LMs protrude into the uterine cavity and, in the same time, the depth of myometrial penetration, SIS provides information analogue to that from the combined use of hysteroscopy and TVUS[13].

In the diagnosis of LM, Stamatopoulos et al. determined MRI sensitivity of 94.1%, specificity of 68.7%, positive predictive value of 95.7% and negative predictive value of 61.1%[14]. MRI has been considered superior to the other techniques in providing exact information about the submucous LMs[7,14-17], but its routine use for all patients is not cost-effective. It is adequate to engage MRI in the patients with high body-mass-index, numerous leiomyomas, very enlarged uterine size, coexistence of LMs and other uterine or pelvic[7]. MRI has been found to have equal specificity, but better sensitivity than US for the diagnosis of adenomyosis/adenomyomas[1,18], which should be distinguished from LMs preoperatively, since the therapeutic strategies differ. MRI with gadolinium contrast represents an appropriate step for preoperative assessment of the likelihood of myometrial malignancy, when US indicates an atypical lesion[5]. Uterine sarcomas in patients undergoing operative hysteroscopy have been reported in 0.13%[19,20].

The use of computerized tomography (CT)[21], virtual CT hysteroscopy[22] and hysterosalpingography[23] is limited in women planning HM, since these do not provide precise information.

Office hysteroscopy allows direct uterine cavity observation, characterization of the endometrium, confirmation of the presence of submucous LMs and other intracavitary pathology. In addition to the direct vision, a biopsy of the endometrium and observed lesions can be performed. Dueholm et al. found hysteroscopy, SIS and MRI to be equally effective and superior to TVUS for the characterization of intracavitary lesions[15]. To correctly define the depth of myometrial penetration, office hysteroscopy should be combined with TVUS. Such a combined diagnostic strategy does not only represent an adequate and recommendable preoperative assessment modality, but also, when feasible, a see-and-treat approach[4].

Recommendation 1: The preoperative evaluation of patients planned to be submitted to HM should start with detailed history and physical examination (Grade 1A).

Recommendation 2: Ultrasonographic examination should be offered to all patients with uterine LMs (Grade 1A) while MUSA terms, definitions and measurements are recommended to be used for the description of scanning and sonographic findings (Grade 1B).

Recommendation 3: For planning HM, evaluation of the uterus with SIS or combined assessment by TVUS and diagnostic hysteroscopy is recommended (Grade 1A). MRI evaluation is appropriate when ultrasound-based assessment faces its limitations (e. g. , patients with high body-mass-index, numerous LMs, very enlarged uterine size, coexistence of LMs and other uterine/pelvic lesions and uncertain nature of the uterine tumor) (Grade 1A).

Recommendation 4: Proper informed consent has to be given to the patient explaining alternative therapeutic strategies, the potential risks of HM, eventual need for a second intervention, and the likelihood of LMrecurrence (Grade1A).

Classification of submucous LMs

Adequate classification of LM is important to guide the treatment choices, including the surgical options. Ricardo Lasmar proposed so called STEPW classification[24], using a score that is assigned on the basis of five submucosal LM features: Size, Topography, Extension of the base, Penetration and lateral Wall position (Table 3). Prospective multicenter studies have demonstrated that the STEPW classification allows a better prediction of complex HM, operative time, incomplete removal of the myoma, fluid balance, probability and severity of complications than the system previously developed by the ESGE does[25,26]. Since HM may require two or more procedures to be accomplished, importantly, the STEPW scoring system is able to predict the risk of surgery in two or more steps better than an estimate based only on LM size and wall penetration[27−29].

Modified from Wamsteker et al. [30], above mentioned ESGE submucosal LM classification includes type 0 (entirely within endometrial cavity), type Ⅰ (with < 50% myometrial extension and < 90-degree angle of myoma surface to uterine wall) and type Ⅱ submucosal LM (with ⩾ 50% myometrial extension and ⩾ 90-degree angle of myoma surface to uterine wall). The classification of the International Federation of Gynecology and Obstetrics (FIGO) uses the same definitions for submucosal LM and includes the categorization of intramural and subserosal LM as well[31].

Recommendation 5: The use of STEPW submucosal LM classification system is recommended to predict the complex surgeries, incomplete removal of the LM, long operative time, fluid overload and other major complications (grade 1B).

Table 3

STEPW classification system of submucosal LMs [adapted from (24)].

Points	Size	Topography	Extension of the base	Penetration	Lateral wall
0	<2 cm	Low	<1/3	0	+1
1	2.5 cm	Middle	1/3−2/3	<50%	
2	>5 cm	Upper	>2/3	>50%	
Score	____ +	____ +	____ +	____ +	____
Score 0−4	Group Ⅰ	Low complexity HM			
Score 5−6	Group Ⅱ	High complexity HM, two-step HM, GnRH agonist use			
Score 7−9	Group Ⅲ	An alternative to HM to be considered			

Abbreviation: GnRH, gonadotropin-releasing hormone; HM, hysteroscopic myomectomy; LMs, leiomyomas.

Preoperative medical treatment

Gonadotropin-releasing hormone analogues (GnRH-a) have been preoperatively used to decrease the LM size and vascularization with the aim of making surgery faster[32,33]. They induce a state of hypoestrogenism that shrinks LMs, but also has side effects such as hot flushes and night sweats. These compounds are combined with hormonal add-back therapy to minimize the resultant hypoestrogenic side effects, including bone loss[34]. In a recent systematic review and meta-analysis focused on the preoperative use of GnRH-a, following outcomes were studied: complete resection of submucous LMs, operative time, fluid absorption and complications such as excessive intraoperative bleeding, uterine perforation and bowel injury[32]. No advantage of administering GnRH-a before HM has been found.

Low-quality evidence exists on the impact of ulipristal acetate (UPA) treatment before HM[35]. The LM treatment by UPA was suspended throughout the European Union pending the completion of an ongoing review of its hepatotoxicity by the European Medicines Agency (EMA)[36]. On 12 November 2020, EMA's human medicines committee (CHMP) recommended restrictinguse of medicines containing ulipristal acetate 5 mg. The medicines must not be used for controlling symptoms of uterine fibroids while awaiting surgical treatment.

Recommendation 6: The preoperative treatment with GnRH analogues is not routinely recommended because it has not been proved to be useful to facilitate a complete resection of submucous LM, reduce operative time and fluid absorption, and avoid major complications (grade 2B).

Type 0 LMs

The key goal of HM is the complete submucous LM removal, respecting the anatomical integrity of the uterus. The operating hysteroscope is the instrument that allows submucous myomectomy under direct and constant visual control. It includes a telescope with final lens ($0°-12°-30°$), an internal and an external sheath of $1-27$ French (Fr) outer diameter that provide a constant inflow and outflow of distension fluid for generating a continuous and efficient lavage system of the uterine cavity. The operating hysteroscope permits the use of working elements: electrosurgical instruments (thermal loops and vaporizing electrodes or laser) and mechanical instruments (scissors, forceps, cold loops) for the traditional resectoscopic or office surgery. Small-diameter office instruments used through the working channel (5 Fr) of standard hysteroscopes ($12-15$ Fr) can be used for removal of small LMs.

Depending on the instrument used, different techniques for hysteroscopic type 0 LM removal are applicable: slicing, morcellation and cutting the pedicle in office setting[4,37]. The classic resectoscopic excision of intracavitary LMs is performed using the slicing technique, which consists of repeated and progressive passages of the cutting loop through the lesion. Excision usually begins at the top of the LM and progresses evenly towards its base. The loop is placed beyond the lesion, while cutting is performed only during the return movement towards the lens.

Although the slicing technique is generally presented as the gold standard for type 0 myomectomy, there is no solid evidence in the literature to support its superiority over other techniques[38]. Intra Uterine Morcellation (IUM) with hysteroscopic tissue removal systems[39], was compared to resectoscopy in a limited number of studies, often conducted on LMs and polyps interchangeably. IUM was demonstrated to be superior in terms of operative time and learning curve. A randomized controlled trial (RCT) reported a shorter learning curve among residents in training for morcellation compared to resectoscopy[40]. A systematic review assessing the feasibility of IUMs in submucous LMs showed positive outcome for type 0 and 1 lesions, unlike type 2 LMs[41]; however, the evidence provided by the studies reviewed in this paper is extremely limited. While IUM is able to remove the submucous LM once it is completely exposed into the uterine cavity, for small pedunculated lesions, office myomectomy can be also considered as an alternative option.

Recommendation 7: For type 0 LMs, in addition to resectoscopy (slicing technique), morcellation is recommended, being faster and having a shorter learning curve with respect to resectoscopy (grade 1C).

Type 1 and 2 LMs

Slicing technique vs. morcellation

Currently, there is a lack of high-quality data indicating the most appropriate technique and instruments for the removal of type 1 or 2 LMs. While slicing technique is feasible and provides reproducible results[1], most of the papers about intrauterine morcellation analyze the technique without discriminating LMs from other intrauterine lesions. In 2017, Vitale et al. did publish a review about hysteroscopic morcellation of submucous LMs[41]. The authors analyzed eight prospective randomized, notrandomized and retrospective studies, but could not provide conclusive information concerning the exclusive use of morcellators for type 1−2 LMs. For this reason, until new good quality studies and data appear, the slicing technique is recommended, because it is practicable and reproducible. At this moment of time, there are no data concerning safety in comparing the two techniques.

Slicing-cold vs. thermal loop

The cold loop slicing technique, first proposed and described by Dr. Ivan Mazzon, has been thought to be less aggressive than thermal loop slicing, in terms of the risk of thermal spreading into the surroundings tissues, i. e. the healthy endometrium and myometrium[42]. However, when performing a myomectomy in the correct plane (pseudocapsula) with a thermal loop, even in the case of a type 2 LM, there should be limited collateral damage.

The main complication to be avoided during myomectomy is the intravasation syndrome. There is no high-quality information in the literature accurately estimating the intravasation rates in patients submitted tomyomectomyaccomplishedbythe cold looptechnique.

Most of the studies focusing the cold loop technique are retrospective or cohort studies, developed by the same group of researchers/surgeons[42,43]. The technique's theoretical superiority with respect to fertility or pregnancy outcome has never been studied in RCTs.

The Mazzon's technique is traditionally performed by the combination of a cold−and monopolar loop[42]. Di Spiezio Sardo et al. published a paper where the technique was used in combination with a bipolar loop[43]. Well-designed randomized trials are needed in order to compare cold loop technique and monopolar/bipolar slicing technique for feasibility, reproducibility and safety.

For above presented set of reasons, no recommendations can be currently formulated concerning cold—or thermal loop's superiority.

Slicing-bipolar vs. monopolar electrosurgery

A sole small RCT was published comparing monopolar with bipolar myomectomy in infertile women with menorrhagia[44]. In both groups, a significant improvement in the menstrual symptoms was observed after myomectomy. Pregnancy-related outcomes were similar as well. In conclusion, there is no proven difference between monopolar and bipolar resection in terms ofthe resolution of symptoms and reproductive outcomes.

Alternative techniques

5.4.1. Hydro-massage and bimanual uterine massage, performed in order to obtain extrusion of the intramural part of the LM into the uterine cavity and reduce, in this manner, the risks of the lesion removal, have been evaluated in a prospective study[45]. This technique could be interesting, but RCTs are necessary to demonstrate its reliability.

5.4.2. Leaving submucous myomas in the uterine cavity after office hysteroscopic enucleation can be an option for small grade $0-1$ LM (1, $2-2$, 5 cm) with 89% success rate, as demonstratedin a small prospective multicenter study by Tanvir et al. Larger studies are needed to establish this technique[46].

Intra-operative ultrasound guidance can be considered. Performed by transabdominal or transrectal probe, in accordance with some authors, it may help to perform the myomectomy in a singlestep and/or avoid complications, such as perforation[47,48].

Recommendation 8: For type $1-2$ LMs, slicing technique is recommended at this moment in time, being feasible and reproducible with respect to morcellation alone (grade 1C).

Recommendation 9: No recommendation can be advanced concerning cold and thermal loop myomectomy for type $1-2$ LMs (grade 2C).

Recommendation 10: Monopolar compared to bipolar type $1-2$ LM resection is equivalent in terms of menstrual symptom relief and reproductive outcome (grade 2B).

Principal HM specific complications and preventive measures

Cervical trauma and cervical/uterine perforation

The complication rates in operative hysteroscopy, Table 4, are mainly dependent on the difficulty of the procedure, the equipment/technique used, the expertise of the surgeon and the characteristics of the patient[49]. About half of all complications are so-called 'entry-related'-cervical trauma and cervical or uterine perforation. Risk factors include anatomical variation (extreme ante-or retroversion) and narrow/stenotic cervical canal due to nulliparity, post-menopause, caesarean section or excision of the transformation zone.

Table 4

Complications of operative hysteroscopy (based on[63]).

Complication	Incidence (%)
Hemorrhage requiring red blood cell transfusion or hemostatic intervention	0.00—0.16
Uterine perforation	0.12—3.00
Infection	0.01—1.42
Operative hysteroscopy intravascular absorption syndrome (using isotonic solutions)	
Mild (absorption of 1000—2000 mL) 5—10%	5.00—10.00
Sever (absorption of > 2000 mL) < 1%	<1
Intrauterine adhesions unknown	Unknown
Resection of multiple vs. singe myomas	45.50 vs. 31.30 *

* Information based on a limited number of cases studied.

Perforation can occur during the cervical dilatation, placement of the hysteroscope/resectoscope or myomectomy itself. A short LM — serosa distance (i. e., myometrial free margin) is an important risk factor. When perforation occurs with an activated electrode, there is a high risk of injury to adjacent anatomical structures. Sometimes thermal injury to adjacent organs may be discovered days after surgery, even without perforation[50].

A conservative approach, with observation and antibiotics, is sufficient in most cases of blunt perforation. However in the case of 'hot loop perforation' a laparoscopic (or laparotomic) exploration is mandatory to fully assess and treat possible damage to adjacent anatomical structures[50].

Different studies give conflicting results regarding the benefit of the vaginal or oral application of misoprostol prior to hysteroscopy, as a ripening agent, to facilitate cervical dilatation and hysteroscope placement[51−53]. Although its use seems promising[51,52], further studies are needed before conclusions can be drawn.

Recommendation 11: The use of vaginal misoprostol prior to HM is not routinely recommended in order to reduce cervical trauma and perforation (grade 2B).

Distention fluid-related complications

To achieve the necessary visualization for diagnosis and treatment of intrauterine pathology the cavity needs to be distended by a medium. During operative hysteroscopy systemic absorption of important volumes of distension solution can occur leading to serious complications (Table 4). The amount of absorption, but also concomitant patient morbidity, such as cardiovascular or renal disease, determine the presenting symptoms and the severity of complications. Fluid overload can lead to heart failure, pulmonary edema, hyponatremia and cerebral edema with seizures, coma and respiratory arrest. The continuous and accurate monitoring of the amount of systemic absorption, the so−called 'fluid deficit', is of the utmost importance for the prevention of complications[54].

Fluid overload with normal saline solution or with hypotonic, nonconductive, low-viscosity fluids (glycine, sorbitol or mannitol) may result, because of supplementary osmotic imbalance, in additional hypoosmolality, hyponatremia and hypokalemia that require multidisciplinary involvement of anesthetists and intensivists in the Intensive Care Unit[55].

Dyrbye et al. found that intravasation exceeding 1000 mL was associated with more extensive gas embolism during bipolar diathermia with saline solution[56]. However, this association is not causal, since the electrons cause the gas bubbles leading to an embolism and not the volume of distention fluid. In bipolar resection, the electrons travel from the active to the passive electrode, just some mm away; the heating of the distension medium is very intense causing "bubbles". In unipolar resection, the electrons travel through the fluid and through the body of the patient causing less heating and hence less "bubbles". Reduced wattage in bipolar resection results in less heating, less "bubble" formation and less embolism in the same amount of intravasated fluid. This is the reason why using small barrel resectoscopes with saline distension medium, with the same wattage, causes the same number of "bubbles" and the same amount of gas embolism as the larger loops.

Furthermore, diathermy produces waste products including carbon monoxide. During HM using bipolar diathermy, carbon monoxide may enter the circulation with fluid intravasation, leading to the formation of carboxyhaemoglobin[57,58]. There is a statistically significant correlation between carboxyhaemoglobin levels and the maximum ST-segment change, also between these levels and the amount of intravasation. This situation can lead to myocardial ischemia. The anesthesiologist must be involved in the complication management. Electrocardiogram changes should prompt discontinuation of the intervention.

Recommendation 12: A fluid deficit of 1000 mL also in case of bipolar myomectomy with saline solution, in healthy women of reproductive age, contains low risk for major complications. Deficits of 1000 mL−2500 mL using saline solution need careful monitoring and termination of surgery at the slightest sign of possible embolism. Deficits of over 2500 mL need immediate termination of surgery (grade 1C).

Recommendation 13: Lower thresholds (750 mL) for fluid deficit should be considered in the elderly and in women with cardiovascular, renal or other co−morbidities (Grade 1B).

Infections

The rate of infection after hysteroscopic surgery appears to be very low (Table 4). No conclusion can be drawn regarding the routine antibiotic prophylaxis until randomized high-powered trialsare conducted in the future[59].

Adhesions

HM can be complicated by postoperative intrauterine adhesions (IUA) of different levels of severity. For this reason, different antiadhesive gels have been developed with the aim of primary prevention. The incidence of postoperative adhesions in patients who have received auto-crosslinked hyaluronic acid gel was reduced versus no treatment group[60,61].

Second look office hysteroscopy is an easy procedure that could be considered, in particular for patients with fertility problems, for diagnosing and removing newly formed IUA[62].

Recommendation 14: Routine hyaluronic acid gel application is recommended after HM, particularly in case of multiple myomectomies (Grade 1B).

Table 5. integrates the information on the studies and sources used to establish and grade the ISGE recommendations.

Table 5

Sources of supporting evidence for the ISGE recommendations.

Recommendations	Information sources (references)
Preoperative evaluation:	
Recommendation 1	1, 4
Recommendation 2	1, 7—10
Recommendation 3	5, 11—13, 15—17
Recommendation 4	1, 4
Classification of submucous leiomyoma:	
Recommendation 5	24—26
Preoperative medical treatment:	
Recommendation 6	32, 33
Hysteroscopic myomectomy—type 0 leiomyomas:	
Recommendation 7	40, 41

续表

Recommendations	Information sources (references)
Hysteroscopic myomectomy—type 1 and 2 leiomyomas:	
Recommendation 8	1, 41
Recommendation 9	42, 43
Recommendation 10	44
Complications and preventive measures:	
Recommendation 11	51—53
Recommendations 12 & 13	54—58
Recommendation 14	60, 61

Note: In the case of meta-analyzes, guidelines and review articles, reference lists of these publications were analyzed and cited relevant papers were assessed.

Conclusions

HM is the most effective conservative minimally invasive gynecologic intervention for submucous LM. The evaluation of the uterus with combined TVUS and diagnostic hysteroscopy or SIS isstrongly recommended as well as the use of STEPW submucosal LM classification system, in order to predict difficult or incomplete surgeries and the likelihood of major complications. For type 0 LMs, in addition to classic resectoscopic slicing technique, morcellation is recommended, being faster and having a shorter learning curve. Instead, for type 1 and 2 LMs, slicing technique is recommended, being more feasible and reproducible with respect to morcellation. The awareness and care to prevent complications are of the utmost importance, in particular, a continuous and accurate measurement of the amount of the absorbed distension-fluid. A fluid deficit of 1 L should be taken as the security limit in all HMs (i. e. , not only during monopolar myomectomy with hypotonic fluids, but also in case of bipolar myomectomy with saline solution) in healthy women of reproductive age. Lower thresholds (750 mL) for fluid deficit should be considered in the elderly and in women with co-morbidities. The evidence-based ISGE recommendations presented here serve to promote patient safety through the promotion of good clinical practice and quality training of the residents.

Declaration of Competing Interest

The authors declare that they have no known competing financial interests or personal relationships that could have appeared to influence the work reported in this paper.

References

[1] Worldwide AAoGLAAMIG. AAGL practice report: practice guidelines for the diagnosis and management of submucous leiomyomas. J Minim Invasive Gynecol, 2012, 19 (2): 152—171.

[2] BONAFEDE M M, POHLMAN S K, MILLER J D, THIEL E, TROEGER K A, MILLER C E. Women with newly diagnosed uterine fibroids: treatment patterns and cost comparison for select treatment options. Popul Health Manag, 2018, 21 (S1): S13—20.

[3] SOLIMAN A M, YANG H, DU E X, KELKAR S S, WINKEL C. The direct and indirect costs of uterine fibroid tumors: a systematic review of the literature between 2000 and 2013. Am J Obstet Gynecol, 2015, 213 (2): 141 —160.

[4] LAGANA A S, ALONSO PACHECO L, TINELLI A, HAIMOVICH S, CARUGNO J, GHEZZI F, et al. Management of asymptomatic submucous Myomas in women of reproductive age: a consensus statement from the global congress on hysteroscopy scientific committee. J Minim Invasive Gynecol, 2019, 26 (3): 381—383.

[5] SIZZI O, MANGANARO L, ROSSETTI A, SALDARI M, FLORIO G, LODDO A, et al. Assessing the risk of laparoscopic morcellation of occult uterine sarcomas during hysterectomy and myomectomy: literature review and the ISGE recommendations. Eur J Obstet Gynecol Reprod Biol, 2018, 220: 30—38.

[6] WHO Guidelines for Screening and Treatment of Precancerous Lesions

for Cervical Cancer Prevention; 2013.

[7] OLALLA S, MONLEON J, CRISTOBAL I, CANETE M L. Diagnostic evaluation of uterine myomas. Eur J Obstet Gynecol Reprod Biol, 2020.

[8] VAN DEN BOSCH T, DUEHOLM M, LEONE F P G, VALENTIN L, RASMUSSEN C K, VOTINO A, et al. Terms, definitions and measurements to describe sonographic features of myometrium and uterine masses: a consensus opinion from the Morphological Uterus Sonographic Assessment (MUSA) group. Ultrasound Obstet Gynecol, 2015, 46 (3): 284−298.

[9] HARMSEN M J, VAN DEN BOSCH T, DE LEEUW R A, DUEHOLM M, EXACOUSTOS C, VALENTIN L, et al. Consensus on revised definitions of morphological uterus sonographic assessment (MUSA) features of adenomyosis: results of a modified Delphi procedure. Ultrasound Obstet Gynecol, 2021.

[10] PEREIRA AEDMM, FRANCO J, MACHADO F S, GEBER S. Accuracy of Transvaginal Ultrasound in the Diagnosis of Intrauterine Lesions. Rev Bras Ginecol Obstet, 2021, 43 (07): 530−534.

[11] FARQUHAR C, EKEROMA A, FURNESS S, ARROLL B. A systematic review of transvaginal ultrasonography, sonohysterography and hysteroscopy for the investigation of abnormal uterine bleeding in premenopausal women. Acta Obstet Gynecol Scand, 2003, 82 (6): 493−504.

[12] BITTENCOURT C A, DOS SANTOS SIMOES R, BERNARDO W M, FUCHS L F P, SOARES JUNIOR J M, PASTORE A R, et al. Accuracy of saline contrast sonohysterography in detection of endometrial polyps and submucosal leiomyomas in women of reproductive age with abnormal uterine bleeding: systematic review and meta-analysis. Ultrasound Obstet Gynecol, 2017, 50 (1): 32−39.

[13] KELTZ M D, GREENE A D, MORRISSEY M B, VEGA M, MOSHIER E. Sonohysterographic predictors of successful hysteroscopic myomectomies. JSLS, 2015, 19 (1): e2014, 00105.

[14] STAMATOPOULOS C P, MIKOS T, GRIMBIZIS G F, DIMITRIADIS A S, EFSTRATIOU I, STAMATOPOULOS P, et al. Value of magnetic

resonance imaging in diagnosis of adenomyosis and myomas of the uterus. J Minim Invasive Gynecol, 2012, 19 (5): 620−626.

[15] DUEHOLM M, LUNDORF E, HANSEN E S, LEDERTOUG S, OLESEN F. Evaluation of the uterine cavity with magnetic resonance imaging, transvaginal sonography, hysterosonographic examination, and diagnostic hysteroscopy. Fertil Steril, 2001, 76 (2): 350−357.

[16] DUEHOLM M, LUNDORF E, HANSEN E S, LEDERTOUG S, OLESEN F. Accuracy of magnetic resonance imaging and transvaginal ultrasonography in the diagnosis, mapping, and measurement of uterine myomas. Am J Obstet Gynecol, 2002, 186 (3): 409−415.

[17] OMARY R A, VASIREDDY S, CHRISMAN H B, RYU R K, PERELES F S, CARR J C, et al. The effect of pelvic MR imaging on the diagnosis and treatment of women with presumed symptomatic uterine fibroids. J Vasc Interv Radiol, 2002, 13 (11): 1149−1153.

[18] AGOSTINHO L, CRUZ R, OSORIO F, ALVES J, SETUBAL A, GUERRA A. MRI for adenomyosis: a pictorial review. Insights Imaging, 2017, 8 (6): 549−556.

[19] VILOS G A, HARDING P G, SUGIMOTO A K, ETTLER H C, BERNIER M J. Hysteroscopic endomyometrial resection of three uterine sarcomas. J Am Assoc Gynecol Laparosc, 2001, 8 (4): 545−551.

[20] VILOS G A, EDRIS F, ABU-RAFEA B, HOLLETT-CAINES J, ETTLER H C, Al-MUBARAK A. Miscellaneous uterine malignant neoplasms detected during hysteroscopic surgery. J Minim Invasive Gynecol, 2009, 16 (3): 318−325.

[21] VILOS G A, ALLAIRE C, LABERGE P Y, LEYLAND N, VILOS A G, MURJI A, et al. The management of uterine leiomyomas. J Obstet Gynaecol Can, 2015, 37 (2): 157−178.

[22] SALEH H S, MADKOUR N M, ABDOU A M, MAHDY E R, SHERIF H E, MOHAMED E A, et al. Role of multidetector computed tomography (CT) virtual hysteroscopy in the evaluation of abnormal uterine bleeding

in reproductive age. Biomed Res Int, 2019, 2019: 1−6.

[23] PREUTTHIPAN S, LINASMITA V. A prospective comparative study between hysterosalpingography and hysteroscopy in the detection of intrauterine pathology in patients with infertility. J Obstet Gynaecol Res, 2003, 29 (1): 33 −37.

[24] LASMAR R B, BARROZO P R M, DIAS R, DE OLIVEIRA M A P. Submucous myomas: a new presurgical classification to evaluate the viability of hysteroscopic surgical treatment. preliminary report. J Minim Invasive Gynecol, 2005, 12 (4): 308−311.

[25] LASMAR R B, XINMEI Z, INDMAN P D, CELESTE R K, DI SPIE-ZIO SARDO A. Feasibility of a new system of classification of submucous myomas: a multicenter study. Fertil Steril, 2011, 95 (6): 2073−2077.

[26] LASMAR R B, LASMAR B P, CELESTE R K, DA ROSA D B, DE-PES D B, LOPES R G C. A new system to classify submucous myomas: a Brazilian multicenter study. J Minim Invasive Gynecol, 2012, 19 (5): 575−580.

[27] MURAKAMI T, HAYASAKA S, TERADA Y, YUKI H, TAMURA M, YOKOMIZO R, et al. Predicting outcome of one-step total hysteroscopic resection of sessile submucous myoma. J Minim Invasive Gynecol, 2008, 15 (1): 74−77.

[28] MAZZON I, FAVILLI A, GRASSO M, HORVATH S, BINI V, DI RENZO G C, et al. Predicting success of single step hysteroscopic myomectomy: a single centre large cohort study of single myomas. Int J Surg, 2015, 22: 10−14.

[29] KESKIN M, ÇAKMAK D, YARCI. GÜRSOY A, ALHAN A, PABUÇCU R, ÇAĞ. LAR G S. Singlestep hysteroscopic myomectomy for submucous leiomyoma. Turk J Obstet Gynecol, 2020, 17 (2): 139−142.

[30] WAMSTEKER K, EMANUEL M H, DE KRUIF J H. Transcervical hysteroscopic resection of submucous fibroids for abnormal uterine bleeding: results regarding the degree of intramural extension. Obstet Gynecol, 1993, 82 (5): 736−740.

［31］MUNRO M G，CRITCHLEY H O，BRODER M S，FRASER I S，DISORDERS FWGOM. FIGO classification system（PALM-COEIN）for causes of abnormal uterine bleeding in nongravid women of reproductive age. Int J Gynaecol Obstet，2011，113（1）：3－13.

［32］CORREA T D，CAETANO I M，SARAIVA P H T，NOVIELLO M B，SANTOS FILHO A S. Use of GnRH analogues in the reduction of submucous fibroid for surgical hysteroscopy：a systematic review and meta-analysis. Rev Bras Ginecol Obstet，2020，42（10）：649－658.

［33］HOSHIAI H，SEKI Y，KUSUMOTO T，KUDOU K，TANIMOTO M. Relugolix for oral treatment of uterine leiomyomas：a dose-finding，randomized，controlled trial. BMC Womens Health，2021，21（1）：375.

［34］ALI M，RASLAN M，CIEBIERA M，ZAReBA K，Al-HENDY A. Current approaches to overcome the side effects of GnRH analogs in the treatment of patients with uterine fibroids. Expert Opin Drug Saf，2021，1－10.

［35］VITALE S G，FERRERO S，CARUSO S，BARRA F，MARIN-BUCK A，VILOS G A，et al. Ulipristal acetate before hysteroscopic myomectomy：a systematic review. Obstet Gynecol Surv，2020，75（2）：127－135.

［36］ROZENBERG S，REVERCEZ P，FASTREZ M，VANDROMME J，BUCELLA D. Suspension of ulipristal acetate for uterine fibroids during ongoing EMA's review of liver injury risk：unfortunate timing during the Covid－19 pandemic！Eur J Obstet Gynecol Reprod Biol，2020，252：300－302.

［37］DI SPIEZIO SARDO A，MAZZON I，BRAMANTE S，BETTOCCHI S，BIFULCO G，GUIDA M，et al. Hysteroscopic myomectomy：a comprehensive review of surgical techniques. Hum Reprod Update，2008（2）：14101－14119.

［38］FRIEDMAN J A，WONG J M K，CHAUDHARI A，TSAI S，MILAD M P. Hysteroscopic myomectomy：a comparison of techniques and review of current evidence in the management of abnormal uterine bleeding. Curr Opin Obstet Gynecol，2018，30（4）：243－251.

［39］EMANUEL M H，WAMSTEKER K. The intra uterine Morcellator：a new hysteroscopic operating technique to remove intrauterine polyps and myomas. J Minim Invasive Gynecol, 2005, 12 (1): 62－66.

[40] VAN DONGEN H, EMANUEL M H, WOLTERBEEK R, TRIMBOS J B, JANSEN F W. Hysteroscopic morcellator for removal of intrauterine polyps and myomas: a randomized controlled pilot study among residents in training. J Minim Invasive Gynecol, 2008, 15 (4): 466－471.

[41] VITALE S G, SAPIA F, RAPISARDA A M C, VALENTI G, SANTANGELO F, ROSSETTI D, et al. Hysteroscopic morcellation of submucous myomas: a systematic review. Biomed Res Int, 2017, 2017: 1－6.

[42] MAZZON I, FAVILLI A, GRASSO M, HORVATH S, DI RENZO G C, GERLI S. Is Cold loop hysteroscopic myomectomy a safe and effective technique for the treatment of submucous myomas with intramural development? A series of 1434 surgical procedures. J Minim Invasive Gynecol, 2015, 22 (5): 792－798.

[43] DI SPIEZIO SARDO A, CALAGNA G, DI CARLO C, GUIDA M, PERINO A, NAPPI C. Cold loops applied to bipolar resectoscope: a safe "one-step" myomectomy for treatment of submucosal myomas with intramural development. J Obstet Gynaecol Res, 2015, 41 (12): 1935－1941.

[44] ROY K K, METTA S, KANSAL Y, KUMAR S, SINGHAL S, VANAMAIL P. A prospective randomized study comparing unipolar versus bipolar hysteroscopic myomectomy in infertile women. J Hum Reprod Sci, 2017, 10 (3): 185－193.

[45] ZAYED M, FOUDA U M, ZAYED S M, ELSETOHY K A, HASHEM A T. Hysteroscopic myomectomy of large submucous myomas in a 1－step procedure using multiple slicing sessions technique. J Minim Invasive Gynecol, 2015, 22 (7): 1196－1202.

[46] TANVIR T, GARZON S, ALONSO PACHECO L, LOPEZ YARTO M, RIOS M, STAMENOV G, et al. Office hysteroscopic myomectomy without myoma extraction: a multicenter prospective study. Eur J Obstet Gynecol Reprod Biol, 2021, 256: 358－363.

[47] KORKMAZER E, TEKIN B, SOLAK N. Ultrasound guidance during hysteroscopic myomectomy in G1 and G2 Submucous Myomas: for a safer one step surgery. Eur J Obstet Gynecol Reprod Biol, 2016, 203: 108－111.

[48] LUDWIN A, LUDWIN I, PITYŃSKI K, BASTA P, BASTA A, BANAS T, et al. Transrectal ultrasound-guided hysteroscopic myomectomy of submucosal myomas with a varying degree of myometrial penetration. J Minim Invasive Gynecol, 2013, 20 (5): 672－685.

[49] MUNRO M G, CHRISTIANSON L A. Complications of hysteroscopic and uterine resectoscopic surgery. Clin Obstet Gynecol, 2015, 58 (4): 765－797.

[50] VILOS G A, ALSHANKITI H, VILOS A G, ASIM ABU-RAFEA B, TERNAMIAN A. Complications associated with monopolar resectoscopic surgery. Facts Views Vis Obgyn, 2020, 12 (1): 47－56.

[51] HUA Y, ZHANG W, HU X, YANG A, ZHU X. The use of misoprostol for cervical priming prior to hysteroscopy: a systematic review and analysis. Drug Des Devel Ther, 2016, 10: 2789－2801.

[52] POLYZOS N P, ZAVOS A, VALACHIS A, DRAGAMESTIANOS C, BLOCKEEL C, STOOP D, et al. Misoprostol prior to hysteroscopy in premenopausal and post-menopausal women: A systematic review and meta-analysis. Hum Reprod Update, 2012, 18 (4): 393－404.

[53] GKROZOU F, KOLIOPOULOS G, VREKOUSSIS T, VALASOULIS G, LAVASIDIS L, NAVROZOGLOU I, et al. A systematic review and meta-analysis of randomized studies comparing misoprostol versus placebo for cervical ripening prior to hysteroscopy. Eur J Obstet Gynecol Reprod Biol, 2011, 158 (1): 17－23.

[54] UMRANIKAR S, CLARK T J, SARIDOGAN E, MILIGKOS D, ARAMBAGE K, TORBE E, et al. BSGE/ESGE guideline on management of fluid distension media in operative hysteroscopy. Gynecol Surg, 2016, 13 (4): 289－303.

[55] LITTA P, LEGGIERI C, CONTE L, DALLA TOFFOLA A,

MULTINU F, ANGIONI S. Monopolar versus bipolar device: safety, feasibility, limits and perioperative complications in performing hysteroscopic myomectomy. Clin Exp Obstet Gynecol, 2014, 41 (3): 335−338.

[56] DYRBYE B A, OVERDIJK L E, VAN KESTEREN P J, DE HAAN P, RIEZEBOS R K, BAKKUM E A, et al. Gas embolism during hysteroscopic surgery using bipolar or monopolar diathermia: a randomized controlled trial. Am J Obstet Gynecol, 2012, 207 (4): 271, e1−6.

[57] FITZGERALD J J, DAVITT J M, FRANK S R, ROBINSON J K. Critically high carboxyhemoglobin level following extensive hysteroscopic myomectomy. J Minim Invasive Gynecol, 2020, 27 (2): 548−550.

[58] OVERDIJK L E, VAN KESTEREN P J, DE HAAN P, SCHELLEKENS N C, DIJKSMAN L M, HOVIUS M C, et al. Carboxyhaemoglobin formation and ECG changes during hysteroscopic surgery, transurethral prostatectomy and tonsillectomy using bipolar diathermy. Anaesthesia, 2015, 70 (3): 296 −303.

[59] MUZII L, DONATO V D, TUCCI C D, PINTO A D, CASCIALLI G, MONTI M, et al. Efficacy of antibiotic prophylaxis for hysteroscopy: a meta-analysis of randomized trials. J Minim Invasive Gynecol, 2020, 27 (1): 29−37.

[60] MAIS V, CIRRONIS M G, PEIRETTI M, FERRUCCI G, COSSU E, MELIS G B. Efficacy of autocrosslinked hyaluronan gel for adhesion prevention in laparoscopy and hysteroscopy: a systematic review and meta-analysis of randomized controlled trials. Eur J Obstet Gynecol Reprod Biol, 2012, 160 (1): 1 −5.

[61] CHENG M, CHANG W H, YANG S T, HUANG H Y, TSUI K H, CHANG C P, et al. Efficacy of applying hyaluronic acid gels in the primary prevention of intrauterine adhesion after hysteroscopic myomectomy: a meta-analysis of randomized controlled trials. Life (Basel), 2020, 10 (11): 285. https: //doi. org/ 10. 3390/life10110285.

[62] SEBBAG L, EVEN M, FAY S, NAOURA I, REVAUX A, CARBONNEL M, et al. Early secondlook hysteroscopy: prevention and treatment of

intrauterine post-surgical adhesions. Front Surg, 2019, 6. https：//doi. org/ 10. 3389/fsurg. 2019. 00050.

[63] AAS-ENG M K, LANGEBREKKE A, HUDELIST G. Complications in operative hysteroscopy：is prevention possible? Acta Obstet Gynecol Scand, 2017, 96 (12)：1399－1403.

图书在版编目（CIP）数据

生育力保护：宫内疾病诊治流程及手术操作规范 /
李雪英主编. — 长沙：湖南科学技术出版社，2023.12
ISBN 978-7-5710-2568-7

Ⅰ．①生… Ⅱ．①李… Ⅲ．①子宫疾病－诊疗②子宫
疾病－妇科外科手术 Ⅳ．①R711.74②R713.4

中国国家版本馆 CIP 数据核字(2023)第 240460 号

SHENGYULI BAOHU —— GONGNEI JIBING ZHENZHI LIUCHENG JI SHOUSHU CAOZUO GUIFAN

生育力保护——宫内疾病诊治流程及手术操作规范

主　　审：冯力民 薛　敏
主　　编：李雪英
出 版 人：潘晓山
责任编辑：王　李
出版发行：湖南科学技术出版社
社　　址：长沙市芙蓉中路一段 416 号泊富国际金融中心
网　　址：http://www.hnstp.com
邮购联系：0731-84375808
印　　刷：湖南省众鑫印务有限公司
（印装质量问题请直接与本厂联系）
厂　　址：湖南省长沙县榔梨街道梨江大道 20 号
邮　　编：410100
版　　次：2023 年 12 月第 1 版
印　　次：2023 年 12 月第 1 次印刷
开　　本：710mm×1000mm　1/16
印　　张：15.5
字　　数：257 千字
书　　号：ISBN 978-7-5710-2568-7
定　　价：88.00 元